CHI KUNG:
WAY OF POWER

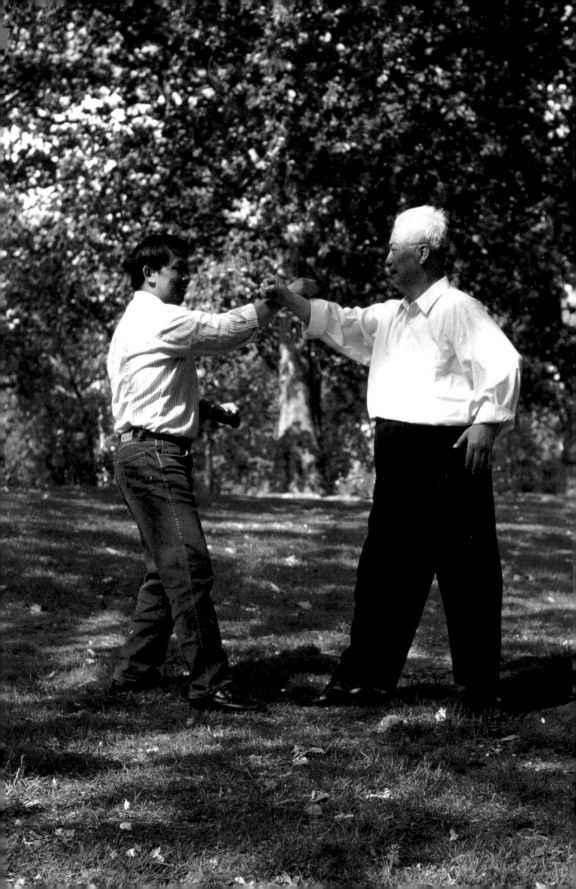

CHI KUNG:
WAY OF POWER

MASTER LAM KAM CHUEN

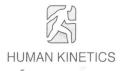

HUMAN KINETICS

Library of Congress Cataloging-in-Publication Data

Lam, Kam Chuen,1950-
   Chi kung : way of power / Lam Kam Chuen.
      p. cm.
   ISBN 0-7360-4480-9
   1. Qi gong. 2. Medicine, Chinese. 3. Exercise--Health aspects/ I.
Title.
   RA781.8 .L36 2003
   613.7'1--dc21

                                        2002009226

ISBN: 0-7360-4480-9

ACQUISITIONS EDITOR: Edward McNeely
ASSISTANT EDITOR: Kim Thoren
INTERIOR DESIGNER AND ILLUSTRATOR: Bridget Morley
COVER DESIGNER: Keith Blomberg
PHOTOGRAPHER (COVER): Paul Forrester
PRINTER: Printed in Singapore by Imago

*Human Kinetics books are available at special discounts for bulk
purchase. Special editions or book excerpts can also be created
to specification. For details, contact the Special Sales Manager
at Human Kinetics.*

10 9 8 7 6 5 4 3 2 1

Human Kinetics
Web site: www.HumanKinetics.com

United States: Human Kinetics
P.O. Box 5076
Champaign, IL 61825-5076
800-747-4457
e-mail: humank@hkusa.com

Canada: Human Kinetics
475 Devonshire Road Unit 100
Windsor, ON N8Y 2L5
800-465-7301 (in Canada only)
e-mail: orders@hkcanada.com

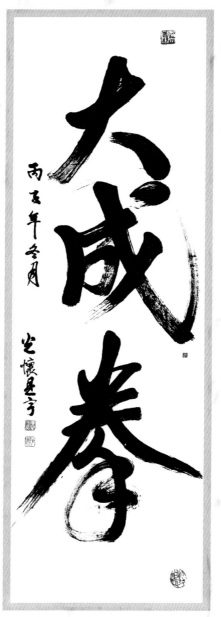

DA CHENG CHUAN
THE GREAT ACCOMPLISHMENT

This book is dedicated to
Grand Master Wang Xiang Zhai,
the founder of the art of
Da Cheng Chuan.

Calligraphy by Master Li Jian Yu,
one of Grand Master Wang's disciples in Beijing.

Contents

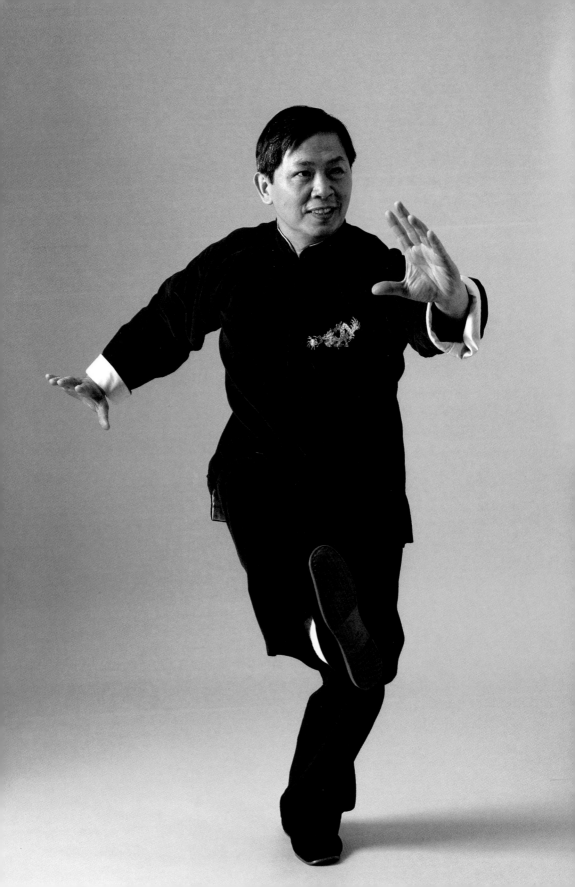

Introduction

All fields of human activity – physical, mental and spiritual – depend on the power of our energy. Properly concentrated, it can generate tremendous creativity and dynamism.

All human beings are capable of manifesting far higher levels of energy than is normally assumed. This book introduces you to the art of awakening this extraordinary capacity already latent in your body and mind.

The techniques for personal development in this book have traditionally been practiced in the martial arts. But the high levels of energy they generate help to transform everyday life. They increase your stamina and brain power. The results work wonders in demanding professions. They give you resilience in high-stress environments and unlock astonishing creative power in the performing arts.

The cultivation of human energy is one of the great achievements of the world's oldest surviving civilization. In the legacy of Chinese culture, the human being is understood to be a field of energy. Natural scientists and medical specialists have worked over the centuries to determine how best to sustain, replenish and enhance this vital energy, known as Chi.

The techniques the Chinese developed for working with our energy are known as Chi Kung, which literally means "internal energy exercise." The most powerful form of Chi Kung begins with energy work involving almost no external movement. This unique system is called Zhan Zhuang, pronounced "jam jong." It is most commonly known as Standing Like a Tree. The stationary postures stabilize the body and unblock the flow of Chi. At a later stage of practice, they can be combined with carefully designed movements to generate remarkable strength.

This seal contains the characters for Zhan Zhuang Kung – The Art of Standing Like a Tree.

Because Chi Kung exercises are so effective in raising our energy levels, they are often used as basic training for martial arts. The practice of Zhan Zhuang is the foundation of one of the most potent martial arts known to the Chinese as Da Cheng Chuan, which means The Great Accomplishment.

Da Cheng Chuan was the crowning achievement of Grand Master Wang Xiang Zhai (pronounced "wang shang jai"), who journeyed for more than ten years throughout China in the first part of the 20th century, studying under the great masters of his day. In the 1920s, he began sharing the fruit of his research with students in Shanghai and later in Beijing.

While there are said to be few, if any, martial arts systems more powerful than Da Cheng Chuan, you experience its enduring benefits as you go about your life and work. Your mind and body become exceptionally alert. Your mental and emotional faculties are refreshed. You experience greater resilience under pressure and recover more easily from illness and injury.

As you work through this book you will find careful instructions, meticulously illustrated. These take you from the first stages of practice through to advanced levels previously unpublished in the West. You will be taught how to employ the Five Energies system in the higher levels of Da Cheng Chuan (see Part Four). You will also learn the way in which precisely controlled movements can be coordinated with essential postures to raise the body's energy to dramatic levels. However, as with all arts, the fundamentals must be understood first and then used as a basis for further achievement.

No matter what level of accomplishment you reach, the energy work in this book will start to generate enhanced inner strength. With careful practice you will be able to use and direct that power in all aspects of your daily life.

The Foundations

If you are completely new to the practice of Zhan Zhuang, it is vital that you first open the gateway to this art. Daily practice is essential, beginning with the three warm-up exercises described below. Then devote yourself to the standing postures on the following pages.

Relaxing the Shoulders

With your feet shoulder width apart, slowly raise your arms as if lifting a ball. Breathe in with the upward movement. Turn your arms outwards and gently lower them back to the start, breathing out. Don't hunch your shoulders or stiffen your arms. Make at least 30 complete circles with your arms.

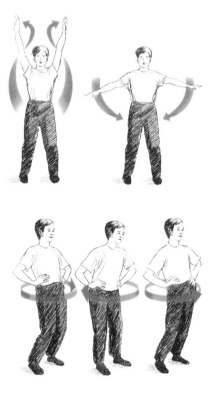

Rotating the Hips

With your feet shoulder width apart, rest your hands on your hips. Slowly rotate your hips 30 times to the left and 30 times to the right. Keep your head gently upright. Let your abdomen soften and your lower back relax. Breathe naturally.

Strengthening the Knees

With your feet together, bend your knees and rest your hands just above them on your thighs. Slowly rotate your knees 30 times to the left and 30 times to the right. Try to keep the soles of your feet flat on the floor. Breathe naturally.

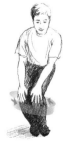

Once you have completed the warm-up exercises, you should undertake the practice of standing still in the following postures. Begin with the first posture, Wu Chi. Stand still in this relaxed position for at least 5 minutes a day, then gradually increase your standing time to 20 minutes.

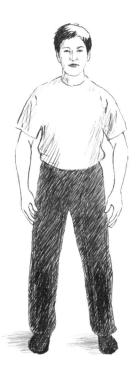

Wu Chi

Stand still with your feet shoulder width apart. Relax your knees, belly and hips. Let your shoulders naturally ease downwards. Your arms hang loosely by your sides. Your fingers are slightly apart, naturally curved. Lower your chin a little and relax your neck. Look forwards and slightly downwards. Breathe calmly through your nose.

This practice is a powerful self-treatment. As you become stable in the Wu Chi posture, your internal energy naturally seeks out accumulated tension and underlying imbalances throughout your system. The detailed instructions on pages 26–27 and the advice on inner strength on pages 34–35 will help you.

Once you have accomplished the practice of standing in Wu Chi for up 20 minutes daily, do the same with the following sequence of positions. Always begin with your warm-ups and an initial 5 minutes of standing in Wu Chi.

1. Holding the Belly

With your feet shoulder width apart, slightly lower yourself as if resting your bottom on a large ball. Bring your hands in front of your lower abdomen as if gently resting a large ball against your belly – or as if you had a very large belly on which your hands are happily resting. Your fingers are gently spread apart and your shoulders completely relaxed.

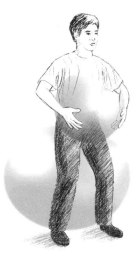

2. Holding the Ball

You continue to sit on an imaginary ball. Your arms form a comfortable circle as if holding a ball between your open palms and your chest. Your elbows sink a little lower than your hands and rest on small imaginary balloons under your arms. Keep your chest and shoulders completely relaxed.

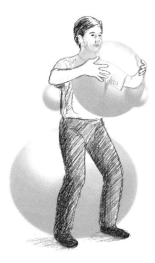

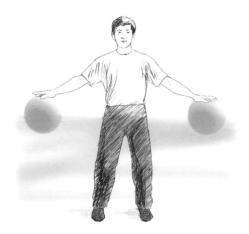

3. Extending to the Sides

Keep the same body posture and extend your arms out to the sides, slightly in front of the line of your body. Relax your shoulders and slightly bend your elbows. You feel as if you are resting your hands on two balloons floating on water.

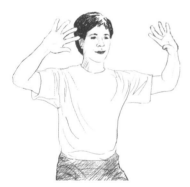

4. Opening Outwards

Open your hands outwards as if pushing a large ball away from your face. Lower yourself a little further, making sure that your knees do not bend forwards over your toes.

Inner Practice

Standing Like a Tree harnesses your internal energy. Stand still, relax, let your central nervous system rebalance itself. Do not add other techniques, such as imagining the movement of Chi around the body or doing special breathing. These can create tension, obstruct the benefits of your practice and do internal harm. The inner work of Zhan Zhuang is uncontrived: be patient, relax, don't move. Your energy will work its wonders naturally.

Sealing your Energy

At the end of every Chi Kung session, it is important to seal into your body the energy you have generated. This applies to the foundation postures and all the positions and movements in the rest of this book.

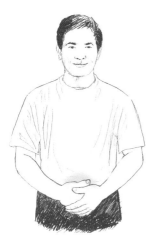

Stand in a relaxed, upright position with your feet shoulder width apart. Place your right palm over your lower abdomen. Then place your left hand comfortably on top of your right. You can lower your eyelids, but keep your eyes open to avoid losing your balance. Rest in this position for between two and five minutes. Breathe naturally.

This position seals your energy into a reservoir just below your navel, known as the Sea of Chi. In Chinese, it is called the Tan Tien (pronounced "dan dyen").

The Mind in your Practice

As you practice the standing postures and movements in this book, your mind is free to roam and experience the thoughts and feelings passing through it. Keep your eyes and ears open to whatever is happening. You can listen to music, even watch television as you practice – flowing music and non-violent channels are preferable. Remain upright, preserving your balance, and devote yourself to the inner relaxation of your being. Everything will flow from that in its own time.

内因是变化的根据，外因是变化的条件，外因通过内因而起作用

矛盾是事物发展的动力

要有基本不动的原则

及以刚柔虚实而静制动

因时起应互错综作用

PART ONE

THE
INNER
DEPTHS

Calligraphy by Grand Master Wang Xiang Zhai,
described in the Introduction to Part One.

Inwardly alert, open, calm.

Outwardly upright, extended, filled with spirit.

This is the foundation of stillness.

Add the hard and the soft, the powerful and the relaxed,

Motion and stillness, contraction and extension:

In the instant these converge, there is power.

The original calligraphy of this poem is reproduced on page 16. The poem is the work of Grand Master Wang Xiang Zhai and takes its place at the very outset of this book because in its few lines are condensed the heart of his instructions to his disciples.

In Part One you are introduced to the standing postures that Grand Master Wang Xiang Zhai taught to his students. They learned the positions after becoming grounded in the foundation postures presented in the Introduction (pages 11–15). Becoming well grounded is the first step in practicing this art.

As you practice standing in the postures of Zhan Zhuang, you begin to experience for yourself the qualities described by Grand Master Wang in his poetry. Your mind becomes more alert. You open up to whatever you experience and your nervous system becomes calm. Your spine is upright, with your body naturally extended from the soles of your feet up to the top of your head. You are highly energized. When you have accomplished the foundation practice, you can then train in the four polarities: "the hard and the soft, the powerful and the relaxed, motion and stillness, contraction and extension." Once you have learned to master these, you reach full strength in body and mind.

Part One teaches you three new warm-up exercises to do before the six advanced standing practices that begin on page 28. The aim of these warm-ups is to relax your major joints, release the tension from your vital organs and open your energy pathways. Always begin with these warm-ups.

To get the maximum benefit from this art, try practicing regularly, daily if possible. To begin with, you might do only ten minutes a day. Gradually, as your practice deepens and you begin to feel its impressive benefits, you will naturally devote more time to your training. Morning practice before breakfast is best; before dinner or bedtime is fine, but never immediately after meals. Try practicing outdoors in the fresh air; if indoors, then open a window. Wear loose, comfortable clothing. You may sweat as your energy expels impurities through your pores. Be sure to rub yourself down after training to clean the residue off your skin.

The essence of this practice and the deep source of its power is the internal relaxation emphasized by Grand Master Wang Xiang Zhai. You should regard the relaxation process described in Part One as the inner work that you need to accomplish in all the postures and movements throughout this book.

As your practice develops try gradually going lower as explained on pages 32–33.

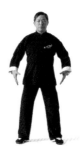

On Guard *Flick through the following pages with your thumb (ending at page 41) to see Master Lam turn to the side and adopt the On Guard position (pages 36–37).* **1**

Opening the Inner Gate

This exercise, Opening the Inner Gate, takes its name from the vital acupuncture point in the center of the lower back. This is one of the most important "Gates of Life" in the human energy structure. The exercise stimulates the Chi throughout your body, releases tension in your hips, torso and shoulders, and massages your internal organs.

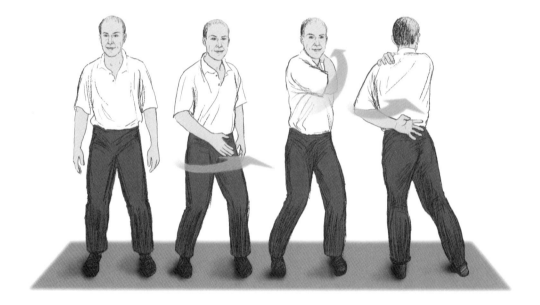

Start with your feet shoulder width apart. Twist your hips to the left, shifting your weight to your left foot and raising your right heel. Do this with enough impetus that your arms swing naturally around with the movement. Your right hand continues the swing up across your chest to slap your left shoulder. Your left hand swings behind your back so that the back of your wrist knocks against the center of your lower back.

Reverse the complete movement to the opposite side. Start gradually until you feel comfortable with the full action. Then develop a continuous motion from side to side, averaging one knock a second. Your shoulders are relaxed. Breathe naturally.

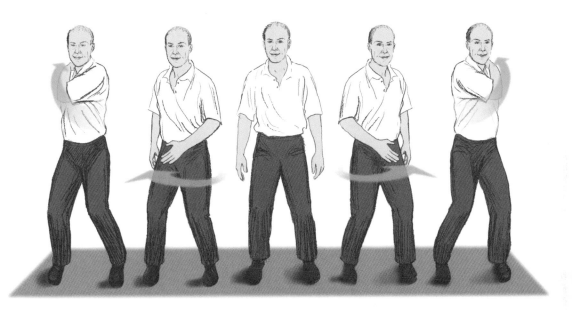

Once you are comfortable with the movements and are able to maintain a completely loose swing, you can take the exercise to the next level. When you shift your weight from side to side, do so with a small bend of the knees. You can develop this into a gentle bouncing on the spot, synchronized with the movement from side to side. Try adding a further bounce as you knock at the gate of life.

Start with 10 complete swings to each side. When you feel comfortable with the movement, you can increase to 30.

2

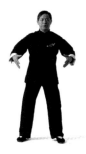

Arm Circles

This exercise releases tension in your shoulders and the upper muscles of your torso. The posture strengthens your Tan Tien and develops power throughout your legs. As your arms rotate like the blades of a propeller, the motion boosts your circulation and extends your Chi from your torso through to your hands.

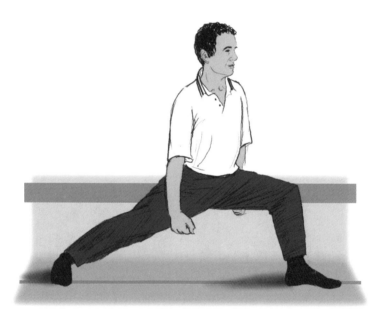

To get into the correct posture, stand with your feet shoulder width apart. Turn your right foot outwards so it points 45 degrees away from the central line of your body. Take a long step forwards with your left foot, so that your stance is as low as you can manage. Gradually increase the depth of your stance as you practice. Your goal is to have the thigh of your forward leg parallel to the ground. Your rear leg is straight, with your foot flat on the floor.

Place your left hand on the top of your thigh where it meets the hip. Make a loose fist with your right hand and swing your arm forwards and around in a full circle. Start with a moderate rate and gradually increase until your arm is rotating as rapidly as possible. Breathe naturally.

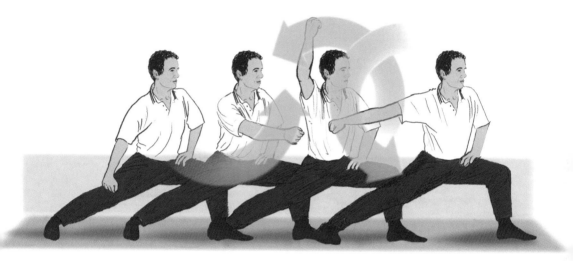

To begin with, go only as low as you can manage. Gradually increase the depth of your stance as you practice. Start with 10 circles using each arm. You can gradually increase to 30. Repeat on the opposite side with your right leg forwards and swinging your left arm.

3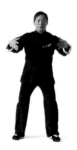

Knees Up

In this exercise you march or run on the spot, with your knees lifted high. It is an instant wake-up call to your cardiovascular system, speeding your circulation and stimulating your breathing. It also promotes your digestion.

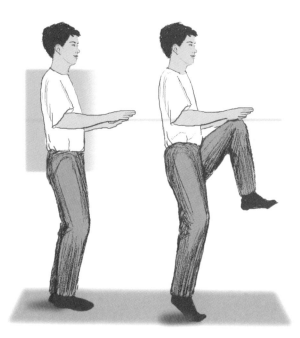

Stand with your feet shoulder width apart. Position your hands in front of your body so that your fingertips are at least 30 cm (1 ft) away from you. Your hands should be level with your solar plexus (the half way point of your torso), with palms face down.

First level (not shown) Raise your left leg until your knee touches your left hand. Lower your leg and then raise the other to the same height, touching your right palm. Repeat, gradually increasing your speed. Then lift your legs with sufficient power to make a slapping sound as they hit your stationary palms. Breathe naturally.

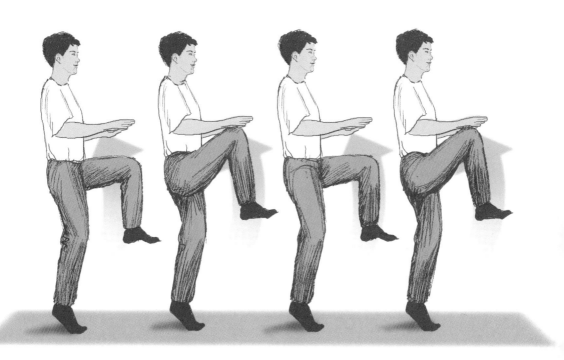

To begin with, do only as many of the knees-up movements as you can. Start with raising each leg 10 times. If you are able, you can gradually increase the number up to 30.

Second level You can increase the power of this exercise by making the same movement while running on the spot, as shown in the drawings.

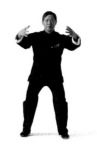

4

Wu Chi

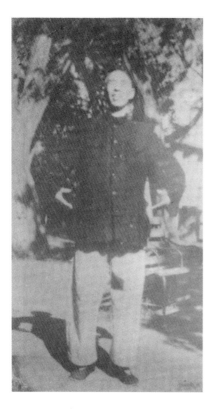

This standing position is known as the position of primal energy. It is the bedrock of Da Cheng Chuan. The Chinese term, Wu Chi, describes the full power of the human being and of the entire universe.

Whatever level of training or personal accomplishment you have reached, your practice should always begin with Wu Chi. This ensures that you are properly aligned, inwardly relaxed and connected to the great sources of power known in Chinese as Heaven and Earth.

As described in Grand Master Wang Xiang Zhai's poem in the Introduction to this part of the book, there is an inner and an outer aspect to this practice. Ensure you are standing in the correct posture and remain completely still. Then work carefully through your body to release any accumulated tension in your muscles. You can guide yourself through this progressive relaxation using the outline on the facing page.

As your practice deepens, you develop greater sensitivity and awareness. You are open to the natural environment and to the constant play of energy around you. In this very old photo of Grand Master Wang, you can see the joyful quality of his practice. You begin to feel the immensity of the earth under foot and the limitless cosmos above. Sometimes, as you stand in Wu Chi, the spontaneous flow of your Chi slowly causes your arms to rise, as if a large balloon was being inflated under them – you can see this happening to Grand Master Wang.

Your head is lightly suspended, as if by a golden cord. Look gently forwards, relaxing your eyes.

Relax your jaw, neck and shoulders.

Imagine water pouring down you, dissolving all your stiffness.

Your arms curve gracefully away from your body.

Gently open your fingers; let them point loosely downwards.

As you relax inwardly, your breathing naturally deepens.

The muscles of your knees naturally unlock; you sink a little, as if about to sit.

Your feet take the full weight of your body, like the base of a great pyramid.

5

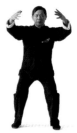

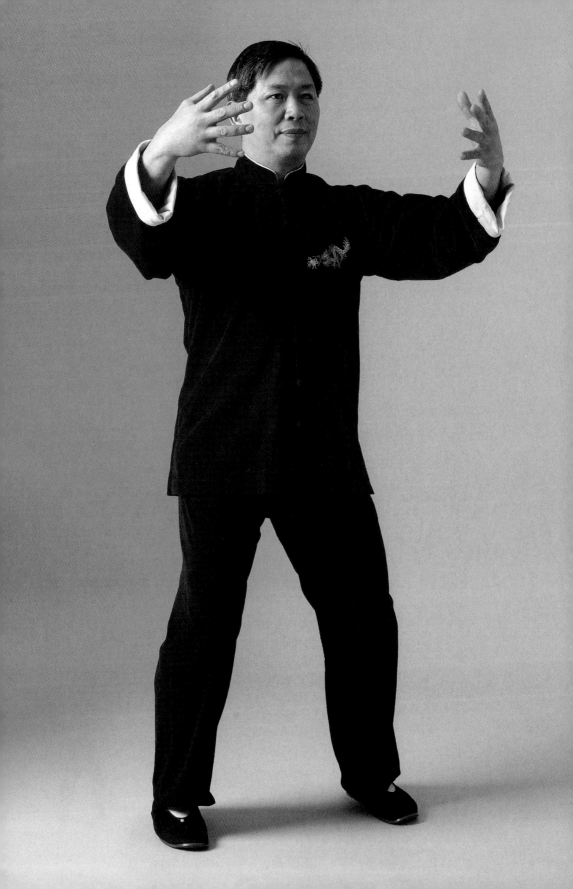

The Great Circle

Once you are thoroughly familiar with the fundamental postures presented in the Introduction (pages 11–15) and are able to stand in each of them for at least 20 minutes, you can begin practicing The Great Circle.

Start by standing in Wu Chi. Then imagine that you are lowering yourself to sit on a large ball. Sink down about 5 cm (2 in). Keep your weight evenly spread over your feet. Do not let your knees bend forwards over your toes.

Slowly raise your arms into the posture, Holding the Ball (page 13), and rest in that position for a minute, ensuring that your shoulders, chest and elbows are relaxed.

Then gradually raise your arms until your middle fingers are level with your eyeballs. As you do this, be careful not to hunch your shoulders or tighten the muscles in your chest or upper arms. You should feel as if your arms floated up naturally.

Allow the distance between the fingertips of your two hands to increase slightly to approximately the width of your shoulders. Your fingers should be gently opened so that there is space between each of them. Your thumbs should be slightly raised, but not tense.

As you hold this position, feel the relaxed curve of a large open circle from your fingertips down to your toes. Keep your eyes open and breathe naturally through your nose. This position is much more powerful than anything you have practiced before and takes time to perfect. Your shoulders or arms may tire after a very short period. You may experience new sensations of tingling, numbness or spontaneous shaking. Allow these feelings to arise naturally. Carefully return to Wu Chi and completely rest in that position for a couple of minutes.

6

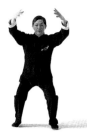

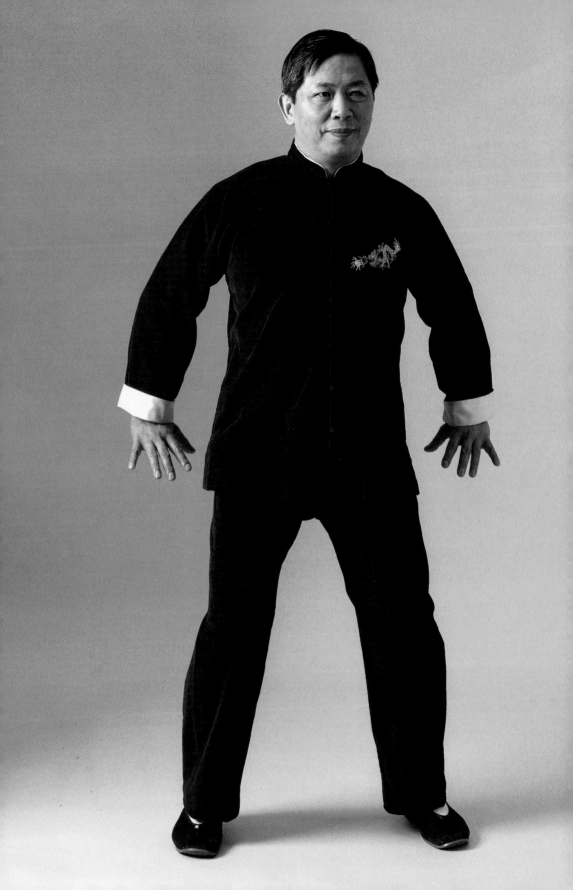

Double Spirals

This position activates two spirals of energy in the body. They coil through and around your arms and hands. You will feel their power thundering down through your Tan Tien into the ground.

You should undertake this exercise only after you have become completely stable in the fundamental postures (pages 11–15) and The Great Circle (pages 28–29).

Start by standing in Wu Chi for a couple of minutes and then The Great Circle for at least five minutes.

Without changing the position of your body, slowly lower your hands completely down and then bring them up behind you as far as you can manage. Keep them away from your body so that they are never hidden behind your back.

Then carefully turn both hands inwards, as if you were trying to get the fingers of each hand to point towards the other. Keep the fingers of both hands open, with as much space between them as possible.

You are likely to feel some tightening in the muscles of your shoulders and your arms. Relax your shoulders by lowering them. Release the tension in your arms by feeling that they are extending outwards to the sides.

It is possible that you will experience some involuntary shaking of the arms or hands at some point while training in this position. Continue to hold your posture calmly while allowing this natural reaction to run its course. You may also find a similar reaction taking place in your legs and abdomen. Again, allow these surges of energy to happen without resisting or exaggerating them. When you tire, which may be after a very short period, slowly lower your arms and return to Wu Chi.

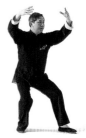

7

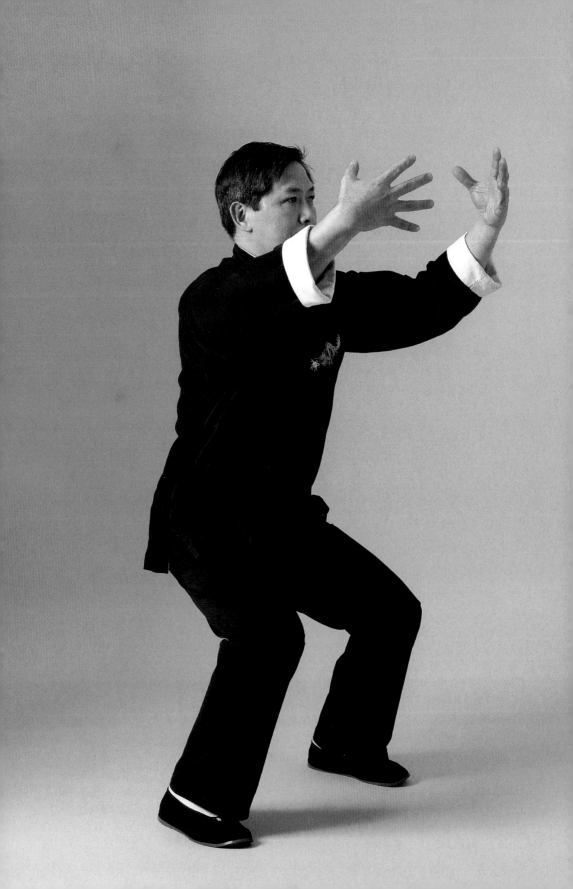

Deep Power

After you become familiar with The Great Circle and are able to remain relaxed in that posture for at least 20 minutes, you can practice sinking lower. Your power deepens as you feel your lower back sliding downwards. Remember to keep your knees from bending over your toes. A slight forward incline of your torso is natural.

Your internal sensations will intensify. Your pulse will probably increase and your breathing deepen. Greater internal heat will be generated and you may sweat.

Despite the effort, keep your mind on the relaxed sensation of holding the large imaginary balloon. Be aware of the spacious-ness between your arms and your body, and also under your elbows and armpits.

Check that your chest and shoulders are relaxed. You may have unconsciously raised your shoulders or tightened your chest when moving into the lower position. Let your shoulders sink down. Make sure your chin is not protruding forwards.

You will find it useful to imagine that you are holding a medium-sized ball between your knees. This keeps your knees from bowing outwards, helps release tension in your hips and lower back, and promotes the correct flow of Chi in the body.

When you have gone as low as you possibly can with your feet shoulder width apart, you can try placing your feet wider apart in order to allow you to go lower.

The inner work of this exercise is simply to maintain the posture for as long as you can. At first, you may only be able to stay down for less than a minute. Don't be discouraged: this deep training requires time for inner transformation.

8

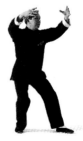

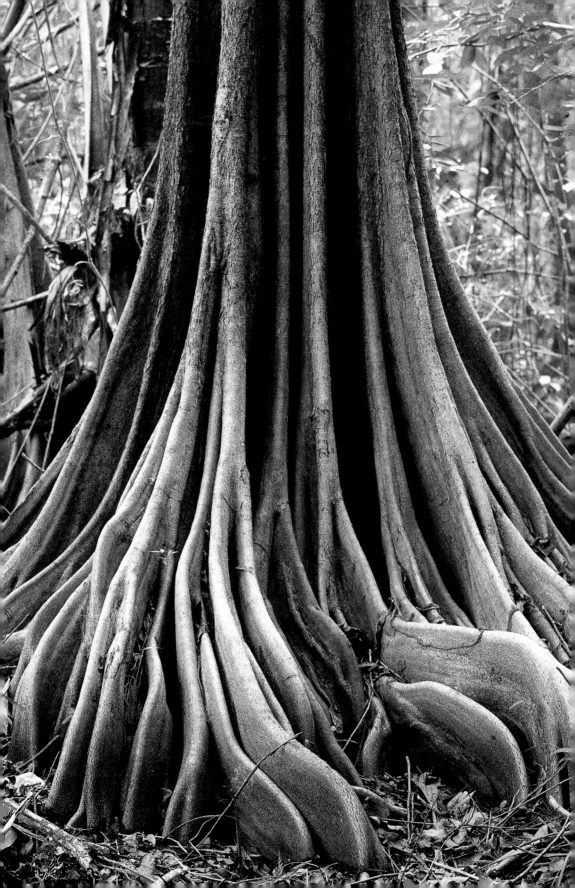

Inner Strength

A mighty tree is deeply rooted in the earth. Its foundations are unseen. It draws its power from the soil from which its seed first grew.

Rising upwards to the heavens, the tree's great mass is still. Countless creatures move across its surface, but the sturdy trunk is calm. It is silent and unmoved, filled with energy.

From its tiny root hairs in the earth to the buds and blossoms far above, the inner power of the tree is circulating, day and night, and season after season.

Feeling wind and rain, and stretching to the light, its delicate, innumerable leaves breathe freely in the energy of space.

This is the inner strength of Standing Like a Tree. Beneath you is the earth, a sphere of power, fertile and immense. It sustains all living beings, as we rest and feed and grow. As you stand and gently soften, inwardly relaxed, the earth's great power feeds your energy.

Above us, expanding without limit, is the galaxy in which we live. Its energy is spinning in a universe of vast, immeasurable power. As we stand, relaxed and vertical, our brain, our senses and our vital organs begin to open, like blossoms in the light.

"To know the riches of the martial arts begin by standing still," Grand Master Wang Xiang Zhai once wrote. "The foundation is Zhan Zhuang – the practice that refines the flow of energy throughout the human body. Zhan Zhuang transforms the weak into the strong and makes the awkward agile. Stand without moving – each of your cells will work and grow. Your blood will move at full capacity and bring your vital functions into harmony. You stand in stillness, apparently inert. Within your being, you are filled with strength."

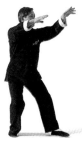

9

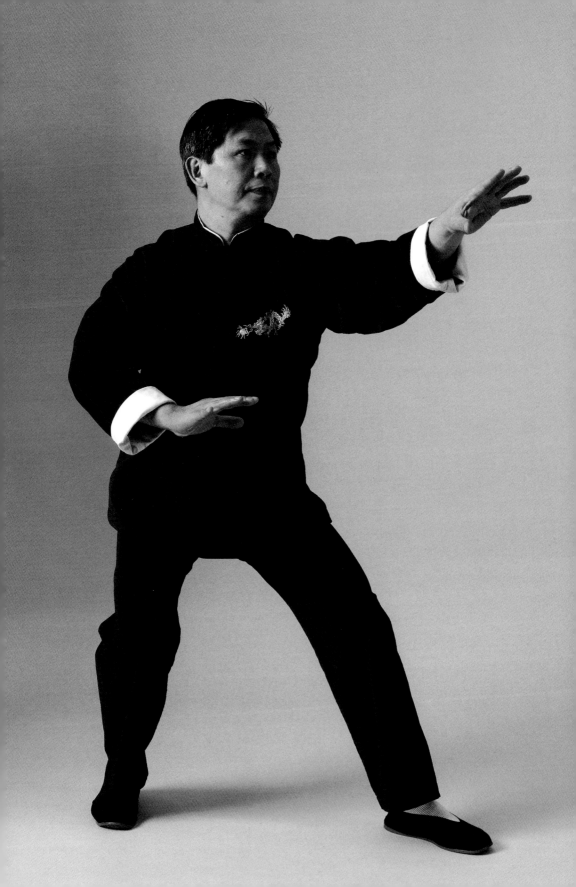

On Guard

You have learned how to root your power in both feet. You now advance to develop the same strength on one leg. This improves your balance and increases your ability to control subtle adjustments in your muscles and tendons. It is the essential foundation for the movements you will learn later in this book.

The preparation for working on one leg is to hold each of the foundation postures with your weight shifted first to one side, then the other. You need to be accomplished in this practice so that you can hold any position with the weight on one side for as long as you normally stand with your weight evenly spread.

To advance to the position shown here, begin in the posture, Holding the Ball (page 13). Shift your weight on to your right foot. Turn your hips and torso slowly to the left diagonal. At the same time, swivel your left foot on the heel to point to the same diagonal. Let your head and eyes turn with your body.

After the swivel, lift your left heel slightly off the ground, as if allowing a little pencil to roll under it. Keep the toes and ball of the foot in contact with the ground.

Lower your right hand until it is level with your navel. Your palm is facing downwards. Turn your left hand so that it extends towards the left diagonal in line with your left toes. This palm also faces downwards.

Relax your neck and your shoulders. Imagine there are balloons supporting you under your armpits and elbows, and a large one on which you rest your bottom.

Train with your body oriented to the right diagonal as well as to the left. As you become familiar with standing in this posture, extend your front foot forwards and sink lower on the back leg to deepen your stance.

10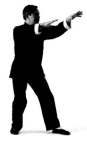

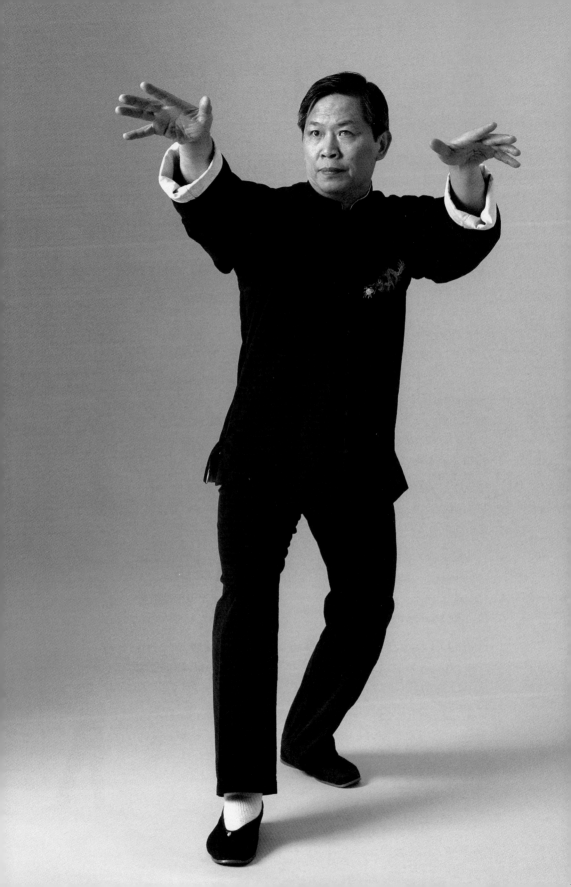

Dragon Mouth

This exercise takes its name from the expressive power of the extended thumb and forefinger on each hand. As the thumb and forefinger stretch apart, they create an energy field like the fully opened jaws of a dragon.

First move into the On Guard position (pages 36–37) and hold it for several minutes to stabilize yourself.

Then slowly sink lower on your rear leg. As you sink, raise both your hands in front of you until they are level with your eyes. Both your arms now extend forwards from your shoulders in the same direction as your front foot. Remember to keep the heel of your front foot slightly off the ground.

Spread the thumbs and forefingers of both hands as far apart as possible. Feel the stretch along their entire length, and the curved web of skin between them. Imagine that the central point between the thumb and forefinger on each hand is directed straight ahead. From this central point, the coiled power of the dragon's tongue is preparing to strike.

Open your eyes and stare intently forwards – in the direction of the dragon's energy.

Once you are able to hold this position for several minutes, slide your front foot forwards on the ball as far as you can until you are as low as possible. Keep your arms in position with the drag-on mouth fully open on both hands. Slightly extend your front knee forwards, while sinking a little deeper on your rear leg. You feel the stretch along the tendons of your inner thighs, known in Chinese as the Kwa.

Hold the position for as long as you can, beginning with very short periods and slowly developing your practice.

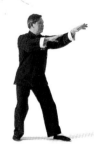

11

Your Natural Strength: Stress Management

Stress is affecting the lives of an ever-increasing number of people. We carry tension with us in our nervous systems and lock it into the cellular memories of our muscles. This strain is the greatest single cause of the headaches, muscle pains, illnesses and medical traumas that people suffer day after day.

In Chinese medicine, health depends on the smooth flow of Chi. Anything which blocks the flow of our energy leads to pain, deterioration and disease. The most common causes of blocked energy are mental and emotional tension.

The foundation postures of Da Cheng Chuan (pages 11–15) develop your capacity to remain calm and relaxed under pressure, and you can use this power to release the effects of stress.

Daily training gives you a high degree of physical and mental stamina. You learn to hold the stationary positions even when your nervous system is rebelling at the lack of movement. You quietly persist despite bouts of impatience, irritation, boredom, panic, fear and anxiety. You develop the physical endurance to hold positions that are often uncomfortable and can be painful, even disorienting. You learn to release the tension through powerful relaxation rather than increase it by fighting back.

Your nervous system develops a new strength. Not the rigid strength of unyielding determination, but the deeper power of inner resilience. You notice a spontaneous equilibrium that persists in the face of difficulties, intense emotions, disturbing environments and discomfort. The advanced levels of Da Cheng Chuan training, which include the martial aspect of this art, further strengthen the field of your psychic energy, increase your endurance and develop fearlessness.

You can use your training to counteract the effects of stressful situations. When you feel stressed, sit up or stand for a few minutes, gently straightening your spine. Let your center of gravity sink downwards. Relax your shoulders. If you are sitting in a meeting, imperceptibly rest your hands a fraction of an inch above your thighs, thus doing a little secret, impromptu Zhan Zhuang practice. If you work at a computer, take a break on the spot: sit up, eyes slightly downwards, hands resting just above your desk.

In difficult encounters with people or in pressured environments, adopt a stable, correctly aligned posture. Use your mind to practice inner relaxation, releasing tension in your shoulders, back and belly. Visualize your body as being like a large tree, mountain or pyramid, with a firm, heavy base – enduringly unshaken through all conditions. The winds of impatience, anger or fear blow across you like passing storms. The power of your inner work will not only protect you in the midst of stress, it will also subtly generate positive energy that changes

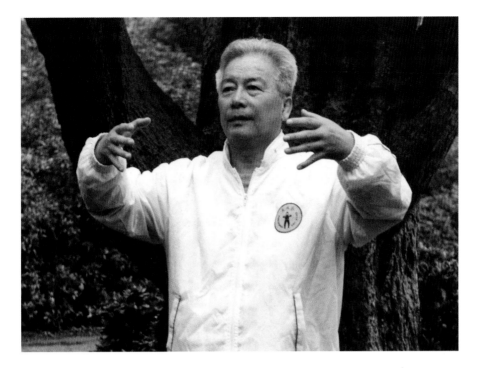

the atmosphere around you. The calming power of Zhan Zhuang seems to radiate even from the photgraph above, which shows my own master, Professor Yu Yong Nian, practicing while on a visit to an English woodland.

When you feel the need to calm down, recharge your batteries or deal with intense emotions, practice Sealing your Energy (page 15) with your hands folded over your belly. Your training subtly transforms your spirit, giving you the inner strength to preserve your vital energy even amidst chaos and conflict.

It is helpful to recall the ancient origins of this art and the extraordinary beings who inspired it. In the words of the great Chinese sage Lao Tse:

There is great danger in pushing forwards relentlessly.
If energy is used to excess, exhaustion follows.
This is not the Way.
Whatever goes against the Way ceases to live.

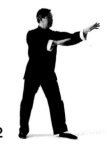

12

THE GREAT ACCOMPLISHMENT LINEAGE I

The practice of cultivating human energy has been passed from master to student in a lineage that stretches over some 27 centuries. The Chinese Philosopher Guan Tse perceived the fundamental nature of energy and saw it as the precondition for all else in the universe. In his writings on the "Natural Way of Life," which he referred to as Tao, he brought together the natural sciences, agriculture, geography, economics, law and astrology. He stressed the fundamental importance of vital power (Jing) as the precondition for all human activity. He wrote: "In order to do anything in this life, we must first have energy."

The great sage Lao Tse (whose name means literally Old Master) is said to have been the author of the Tao Teh Ching, one of the most widely read and influential books in the course of human civilization. It says: "By standing alone and unchanging, you will find that everything comes to you and the energy of the cosmos will never be exhausted." "Standing alone and unchanging" was his way of describing the practice through which we come to understand the full power of the universe.

The world's most influential medical text, *The Yellow Emperor's Classic of Internal Medicine* (*Huang Ti Nei Ching*), appeared some 2,400 years ago. It is filled with references to the essential spirit of this tradition. The court physician tells the Emperor: "The sages were tranquilly content with nothingness and the true vital force accompanied them always. Their vital spirit was preserved within..."

In the works of the Taoist philosopher Chuang Tse there is a chapter on "The Great and Most Honored Master," which expresses many of the essential qualities inherent in the practice of Zhan Zhuang. Chuang Tse tells us that the sages of

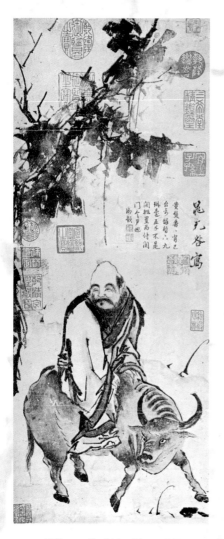

Silk scroll of Lao Tse, with imperial seals.

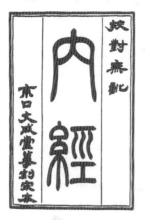

*The cover of The Yellow Emperor's
Classic of Internal Medicine*

old were "still and unmoved." "Their breathing came deep and silent" and their "minds were free from all disturbance," "forgetting everything." They were "open to everything and forgot all fear of death."

A disciple tells his master, "I am making progress." "What do you mean?" asks the master. "I sit and forget everything... becoming one with the great void in which there is no obstruction."

In the 1st century CE, exercises for the cultivation of internal energy (Chi) were developed as part of Taoism and included the practice of remaining completely still in fixed positions. Emphasis was then placed on using the mind to control the movement of internal energy within the body and then to project it outwards.

Buddhist thought and practice also had an influence on the development of the tradition. When the Buddhist practice of "one-pointedness" of mind (the ability to focus the mind clearly) was incorporated into Chi Kung training, mental concentration could be used to help cultivate Chi energy throughout the body and direct its movement.

From the 12th century CE onwards this understanding of energy and the intimate body/mind relationship was employed in the progressive deepening of the internal martial arts.

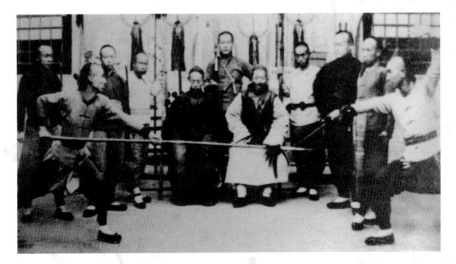

A martial arts academy in 1911 is presided over by Master Guo Yun Sin (seated in white), under whom Wang Xiang Zhai studied.

獨立守神

錦全同學

師永年

九三年四月

THE WELL-TEMPERED SPIRIT

Calligraphy by Professor Yu Yong Nian,
described in the Introduction to Part Two.

Stand still, keep your spirit.

The original calligraphy of this epigram is reproduced on the opening page of Part Two (page 44). It is the work of Professor Yu Yong Nian, my master in Beijing. The complete scroll, from right to left, reads:

To my student Kam Chuen,
"Stand still, keep your spirit,"
your master Yong Nian, April 1993.

The four large central characters are from an ancient Chinese text. The first two literally mean "stand there," with a sense of solitude. They point to the deep stillness of Zhan Zhuang, the practice that is the foundation of Da Cheng Chuan. Zhan Zhuang literally means "standing like a stake" in Chinese. To Western ears the idea of standing like a stake seems lifeless, like dead wood, so we normally use the phrase "standing like a tree," This helps us understand that although we are not moving, we are growing within. Nevertheless, there is great significance in the original Chinese terminology because it directs our mind to the complete and utter stillness of the foundation practice. We train ourselves to rest in the Zhan Zhuang postures without moving at all, yet developing the discipline of deep relaxation.

Speaking to students in Europe on one of his rare trips outside China, Professor Yu told them to persevere with their training: "Stillness is the first step. This opens the door. There are other jewels hidden in the darkness which you will come to understand only through your own practice."

The second two characters of the epigram literally mean "on guard, spirit." In societies where people separate mind and body, the text could be interpreted to mean that our still body is protecting our spirit within. But in the profound tradition of the classical Chinese arts – philosophy, medicine and the martial arts – mind and body are one. Therefore, the stillness to which this epigram refers is the stillness of your whole being. To stand still is to be still; the stillness of your standing is the stillness of your spirit. Just as with great mountains, sturdy trees and an invincible spirit, it is in profound stillness that all power is born.

In one of his most widely read books on Zhan Zhuang, Professor Yu reminds us that what we today call "martial arts" or "the way of the fist" derives from practices that the great sage Guan Tse called "the art of the spirit."

As your training develops in Part Two, you are introduced to progressively more powerful postures. You may feel that you are pushing your body beyond the limits of its endurance. At first, the effort seems almost entirely physical. Then you begin to perceive that it is the entire energy field of your body/mind that is being transformed. In one of his poems, written for the benefit of his disciples, Grand Master Wang Xiang Zhai wrote:

You are going through a furnace:
Everything mental and physical
is being tempered and molded.

Dragon and Tiger *Flick through the following pages with your thumb (ending at page 67) to see Master Lam move from The Dragon position into Holding the Tiger (pages 64–67).* **1**

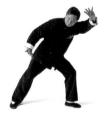

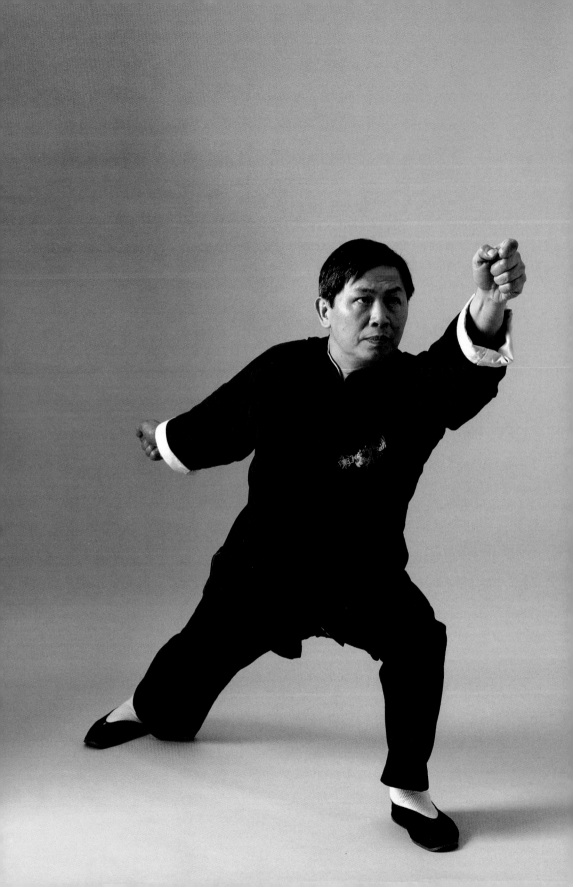

The Archer

This deep posture rapidly extends your Chi from your Tan Tien out to your extremities, thereby increasing its flow throughout your entire system. It is a powerful foundation practice for the martial arts applications of Da Cheng Chuan, and works instantly to make you mentally alert and energized.

You should undertake this practice only after completing the warm-up exercises in Part One (pages 20–25).

The Archer begins in Wu Chi. Your feet are shoulder width apart. Turning to the left, swivel on the heel of your left foot. Your left foot is now at right angles to your right foot. Your head and upper body are turned in the direction of your right foot.

Step forwards with your left foot, making as long a step as possible. Extend your stance by sliding your left foot further forwards. As you practice this posture, your aim will be to extend your stance until your front thigh is parallel with the ground. Your back leg is straightened with your rear foot flat on the floor.

Raise both your arms so that your right arm is pointing straight back over your rear leg and your left arm points straight ahead over your front left leg. Make sure the left hand is slightly higher than the level of your head.

Fold both your hands into loose fists. Connect the pads of your thumbs to the first knuckle of your forefingers. This creates a arrowhead on each fist, as you can see in the photograph.

Maintain this posture for as long as you can. Feel the power surging in your legs and your Tan Tien. Breathe naturally.

Repeat The Archer so that your right foot and arm are pointing forwards, with your left foot and arm to the rear.

2

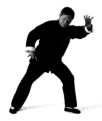

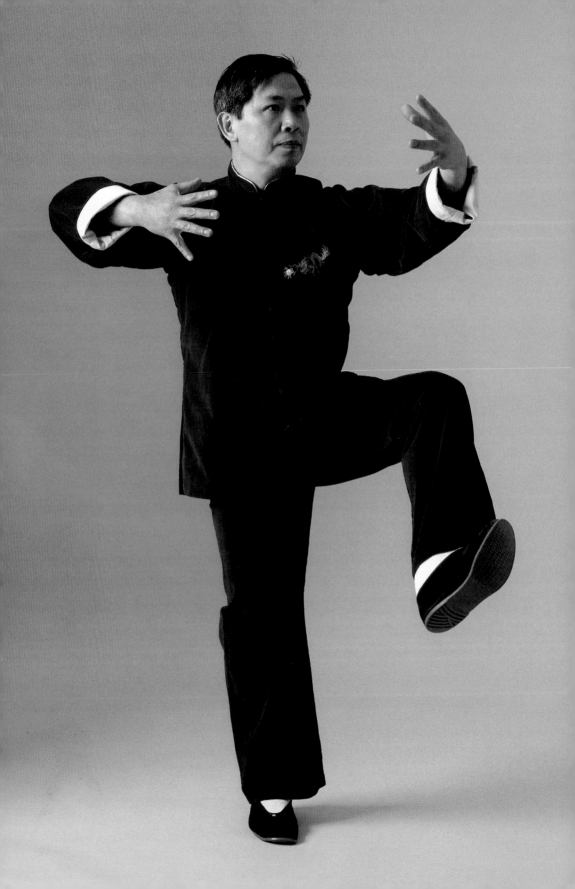

Rising Up

This is the stage at which you start to practice bearing the full weight of your body on one leg. It is essential training for your balance and agility, and for the power that you will be able to generate throughout your entire body.

The first step is to train on one leg, with the other supported. Stand with your feet shoulder width apart about 30 cm (1 ft) in front of a chair or table. Raise your arms into the posture, Holding the Ball (page 13). Swivel your right foot 45 degrees away from the central line of your body. Place the outer side of your left heel on the chair or table. Turn your left foot and knee outwards. Only a fraction of your weight should be on the raised heel. It is only there for balance. Hold that position, first on one leg, then the other, for as long as you normally practice standing with both feet on the ground.

Now you can begin the practice of working fully on one leg. Your rear foot should always be turned 45 degrees outwards. This is for maximum support. Raise your other leg, as if placing it on a chair or table. Stretch your toes upwards as far as you can and turn your raised foot outwards. As you stand, practise sinking your weight fully down through your stationary rear leg. At the same time, you feel your head being lightly held aloft by a golden cord reaching up into the sky. Relax the muscles of your raised leg, just as you did when resting it on a chair or table.

You can practice holding each of the arm positions used in the foundation postures (pages 11–15) while rising up on one leg. Try to hold the position for as long as you possibly can. Examine the ways in which subtle adjustments of your posture can release accumulated strain and help you maintain your balance. This trains your central nervous system.

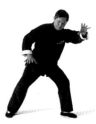

3

Wall of Fire

This exercise is one of the first stages in training your whole body to move as a unit. It enables you to use the full field of your energy without blocking the flow at any of your joints. The skill developed in this way can be applied in many martial arts. This practice strengthens your hands and trains you to use their power with minimal effort.

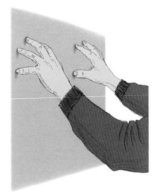

Stand in Wu Chi about 30 cm (1 ft) from a wall. Step back with your left foot, placing it on the ground at a 45-degree angle. Your rear leg is straight and the sole of the foot is flat on the ground. Your front knee is slightly bent so that the lower part of the leg is at right angles to the ground.

Place the fingertips of both your hands on the wall at the level of your shoulders. Spread your fingers apart so that there is a comfortable space between each of them. Make sure the tips of both your thumbs are also touching the wall. Gently curve each finger and thumb as if they were surrounding the surface of a bowl. This naturally causes your palm to curve slightly as well.

Gradually transfer your weight forwards on to your fingertips. This takes the weight off your front foot so that your body is supported by your rear foot and fingertips. As you develop strength, you can lift your front foot slightly off the ground while holding the position.

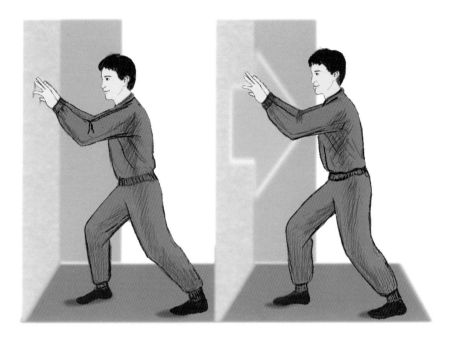

When you have developed the strength and stability to hold this position, you can move to the next level. With both feet on the floor, weight resting on your rear leg and fingertips, breathe in. When you are ready to breathe out, do so while pushing yourself away from the wall using only a slight extension of your fingers.

This little push will move your whole body a short way off the wall. Repeat again and again. Gradually, you will be able to do this while maintaining the curves of your fingers and palms and with almost no effort in your arms, shoulders or chest.

When you have reached this stage of practice, imagine that the wall is burning. It could be a wall of fire or a sheet of metal that is red hot. You want to touch it only for a split second and bounce off it instantly. Breathe out with the same speed.

Repeat this exercise, practicing sometimes with your left foot forwards, sometimes with your right foot forwards.

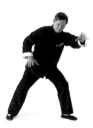

4

Shoulder Strike

This exercise continues to train you to move your body as a unit.
It can be used in the martial arts and also as a protection in the
case of accidents or falls.

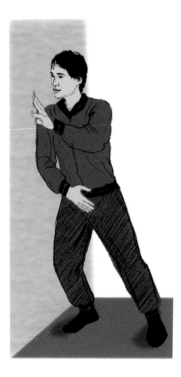

Stand in Wu Chi with a wall on your right
side. You should be at right angles to
the wall, with your right foot no more
than 8 to 10 cm (3 or 4 in) from the wall.

Raise your left hand so that it is in front
of your right shoulder, with the palm
facing the wall. As in the Wall of Fire
exercise (pages 52–53), spread your
fingers and gently curve them as if they
were around a bowl.

Shift your weight to your right side so that your shoulder rests
against the wall. The tips of the fingers and thumb of your left
hand lightly touch the wall. Transfer more weight to your right
side so that your body is supported along a line from your left
foot to your right shoulder. Relax the rest of your body, keeping
the straight line between your foot and shoulder. Try lifting your
right foot slightly off the ground while holding the position.

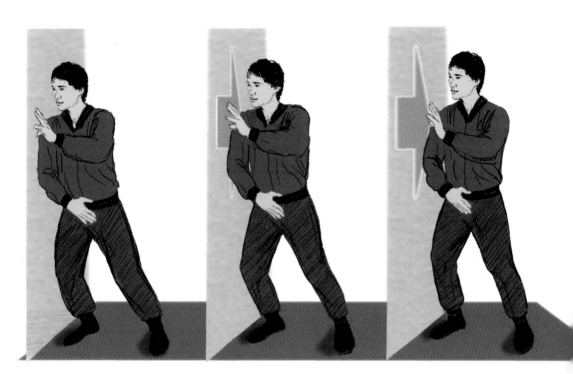

Train in this position until you are able to rest without moving for
several minutes. Then, with both feet on the ground, push yourself away from the wall using both your shoulder and the tips of
your fingers and thumb. Breathe out as you make this move.

This little push will move your whole body a short way off the
wall. Repeat again and again until you are able to bounce back
and forth off the wall. The instant your right shoulder and left
hand make contact with the wall, relax into the contact for a split
second and bounce off instantly. Breathe out each time you
bounce away from the wall.

Repeat this exercise, practicing sometimes with your left
shoulder towards the wall, sometimes with your right.

5

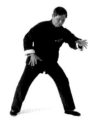

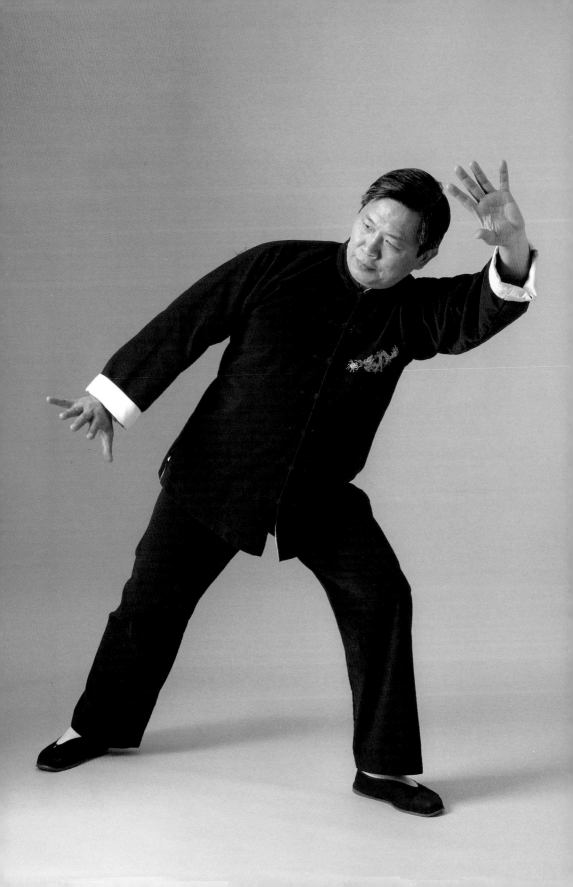

The Dragon

The Dragon position, and the posture that follows it, Holding the Tiger, are suitable only for practitioners who have developed a regular, daily practice and are capable of remaining stable in the postures already introduced in this book.

Before practicing The Dragon, which opens the energy pathway of the spinal column and stimulates your central nervous system, you must do the warm-up exercises that loosen your shoulders, hips and knees (pages 20–25). Then stand in Wu Chi for five minutes, working on inner relaxation and establishing a deep connection with the energy of the earth.

Swivel on your left heel until your toes point 90 degrees to the left. Turn your head to look in that direction.

Step forwards with your left foot, keeping your right foot firmly in place. The lower part of your left leg is perpendicular to the floor. Your right leg will naturally incline in the direction of your left foot and be straight with the foot flat on the floor.

Transfer as much of your weight as you can on to your left leg. Lean your torso over to that side, making a straight line from the outside of your right foot up to your left shoulder.

Raise your left hand up and turn it to press away from your head. Your right hand presses away in the direction of your rear foot. The fingers of both hands are spread apart. Look at the back of your right hand.

Feel the weight of your body balanced on your front foot. This is the point from which the dragon arises from the earth. As you relax, you feel the extension of your body as if you were coiling outwards. Your hands open into the air like the spreading talons of a dragon in space.

6

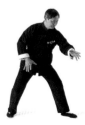

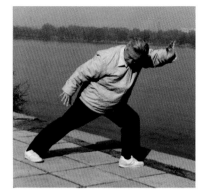

The full title of this posture is The Dragon at Ease. It is the first stage in learning the advanced dragon position, which must be done under the personal guidance of a master or authorized instructor. Since the basic elements of the advanced stage of this position are contained in The Dragon at Ease, it is essential to pay attention to all the details from the very beginning.

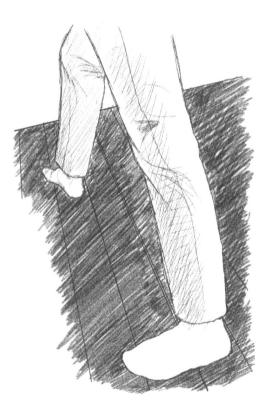

Your feet are at right angles to each other, with the toes of your front foot pointing in the direction in which you are leaning. Your heels are in line with each other. The knee of your front leg does not extend forwards over your toes. Your back leg is straight. The line of your upper body is an extension of the line of your rear leg. You can begin with a moderate stance and gradually extend it until you are much lower, as in The Archer (pages 48–49). Practice also with your left foot forwards and right foot back.

As you lean to one side, more and more of your body weight shifts to your front foot. As this happens, try to keep your forward hand as high as possible. It should be at least as high as your head. Your palm is turned outwards and your fingers are spread apart, like the talons of a dragon. Your rear hand is level with your hips. The palm is turned to press away in the same direction as your rear foot, with the fingers fully spread. Your head is turned so that you can look in the direction of your rear hand.

7

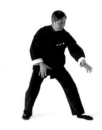

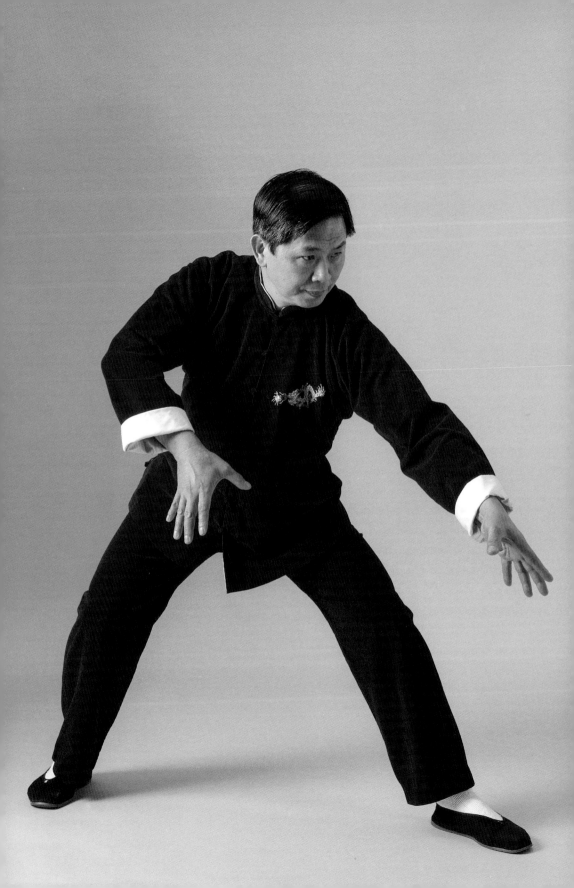

Holding the Tiger

Holding the Tiger is one of the most advanced postures in this entire Zhan Zhuang system. It relaxes your hips and lower back, strengthens the Tan Tien and the Kwa tendons of the inner thighs, and tones the major muscles in your legs.

Begin by standing in Wu Chi for five minutes, relaxing throughout and ensuring that you release any tension in your abdomen, hips and lower back.

Continue by standing in the posture, Holding the Ball (page 13), for a further five minutes. Relax your shoulders and chest, feeling completely supported by the energy around you.

Then turn into the On Guard position (pages 36–37). Settle into this posture, with at least 60 percent of your weight on your rear leg. The ball and toes of your front foot touch the ground, while your heel is slightly raised.

Once you are stable in the On Guard position, slowly incline your torso forwards. Be sure to move your upper body as one unit, keeping the same alignment of your head, shoulders, arms and hands. Continue the incline until your fingers are pointing towards the ground as shown in the picture on the facing page. Adjust your gaze to follow the line of your front hand towards the space ahead of you.

After practicing this first stage, you can enter the position directly from Holding the Ball. Take a large step backwards with one foot, placing it firmly on the ground at a 45-degree angle. Then transfer your weight back to that leg and lower yourself into Holding the Tiger. Your stance will be more extended and deeper. You can use the ball of your front foot to press your weight backwards towards your rear leg.

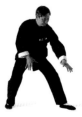

8

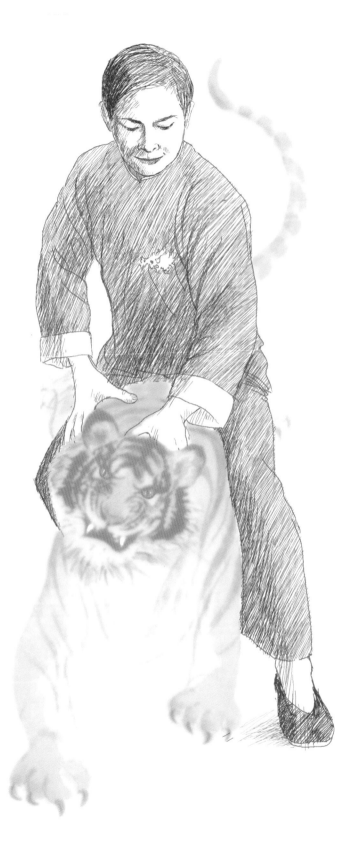

This position, Holding the Tiger, takes its name from the intense energy which it generates. Try to visualize holding the tiger using the picture opposite – it can help you adopt the correct posture (pages 60–61).

Once you have learned the basic positions for your feet and hands and have practiced holding the posture without moving, you can apply your mind to holding the imaginary tiger.

Begin by feeling that you are completely astride the tiger, your feet firmly on the ground. The tiger's body is held in position between your legs so that his long tail and powerful back legs stretch out behind you. His back runs along between your thighs and forwards under your palms. As you look slightly down and forwards, you can see the top of his head just in front of you. Your front hand is placed firmly around the back of his neck, so that his head is under your control.

Feel that you are pinning the tiger down by squeezing his flanks between your knees. This pressure just above his hips deprives his back legs of their power. Let your weight sink downwards so that the tiger's haunches are compressed under the lower end of your spine.

The hand nearest to your belly rests calmly on the tiger's back. Open your forward hand so that you feel as if the broad curve formed by your thumb and forefinger is pressed under the back of the tiger's skull. You use this hand to take control of the upper end of his spinal cord. Constantly check that your upper body and neck remain completely relaxed.

Your gaze should be aimed at the back of the tiger's head, watching his every move. You feel his explosive power coiling underneath you as he tries to shake you off.

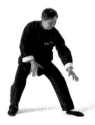

9

Dragon and Tiger

On the next four pages, you will learn how to move between the
two positions you have just learned: The Dragon and Holding the
Tiger. Before attempting to do this, you should have practiced
the two postures thoroughly until you can remain stable and
relaxed in both. Before starting this sequence, you must do
the preliminary exercises that loosen your shoulders, hips and
knees (pages 20–25).

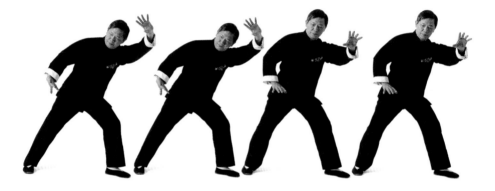

After warming up, stand in Wu Chi, as always. Then progress to
Holding the Ball (page 13) for at least five minutes.

Slowly move into The Dragon posture. Step forwards with your
left foot, keeping your right foot firmly in place.

After remaining in The Dragon posture for a minute, use the
power in your front leg to slowly raise yourself. All the work is
done by your front leg, as if it were a hydraulic pump.

The accomplishment of Da Cheng Chuan results from sustained practice. Day by day your body starts to change. You are training muscles never used before and relaxing those unnecessary for the challenge ahead. Learning the correct postures is the foundation of the powerful movements you will be practicing.

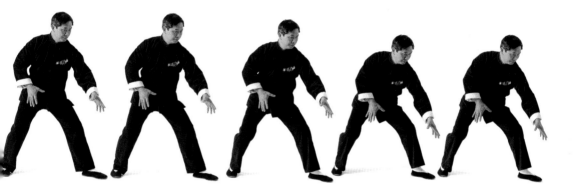

The upward motion slowly shifts your posture gradually backwards until you can lower yourself down over your back leg.

Your hands change into the position for Holding the Tiger.

You complete the posture with your front heel slightly raised and your hands controlling the body of the tiger in front of you.

Breathe naturally through your nose as you move.

10

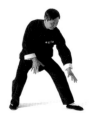

Dragon and Tiger reverse sequence

Once you have practiced moving from The Dragon into Holding
the Tiger, you can then reverse the sequence, as shown below.
Eventually, you can practice moving carefully between the two
positions in a continuous, wave-like flow.

This entire sequence must be done slowly, with careful attention
to the correct progression from posture to posture.

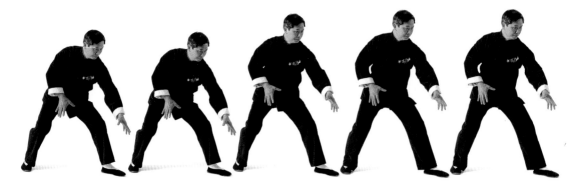

Remain in Holding the Tiger for a few moments to stabilize yourself. Then, using your back leg like a hydraulic pump, gradually
start to come up. The movement of your rear leg gradually starts
to shift your weight forwards. When your weight is distributed
evenly over your feet, begin to move into The Dragon posture.
Your weight transfers as fully as possible on to your front foot.

Your rear leg extends until it is fully straightened. Your torso leans
in the direction of your front foot, so that there is a straight line
from your rear foot up to your shoulder. As you change your
posture, your arms and hand uncoil to the fully extended
Dragon posture.

In the course of his studies, Grand
Master Wang Xiang Zhai delved deeply
into the spiritual heritage of Chinese
culture, immersing himself in the wisdom
of the Taoist and Buddhist traditions.
His insight and his love of the arts are
reflected in the inspiring poems he wrote
for the benefit of his disciples:

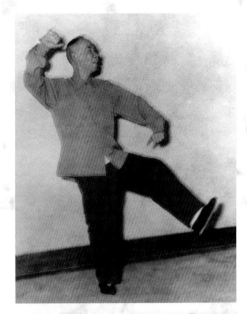

*In quietness you are like a maiden
In motion you are like a dragon.
The mountains seem to fly
when you apply your mind,
The seas overflow
when you apply your power.*

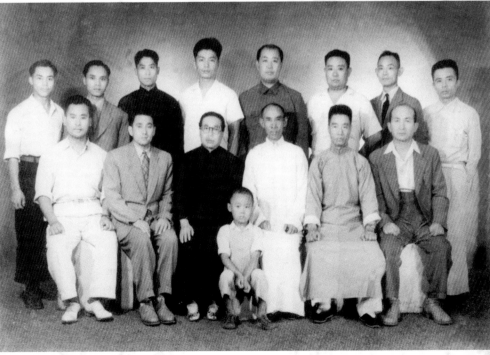

Grand Master Wang Xiang Zhai (in classical white Chinese gown) seated with his students.

渾身肌肉掛青霄　毛髮根根暖風
搖蕩眼默察三千寄擬耳愈聽二人
嬌淪海飛波游龍戲流雲江上月紫兔噴水
無窮假借無窮有如蓬臺踏六鰲

王薌齋恩師遺作也詩詞言拳文筆洒脫抒寫習拳體驗值明之深奧尋味無窮

繼芳先生　雅囑　清鑒
己丑春三月　默々齋主　賴省　孔潤泉

PART THREE

THE
WEB OF
STRENGTH

Calligraphy by Grand Master Wang Xiang Zhai,
described in the Introduction to Part Three.

Within the body the muscles are at ease, suspended from the sky.
Outside, each hair is active, moving with the air.
The inner eye is quiet, seeing the three thousand.
The ear listens intently to its own body, like eavesdropping on lovers.
Play like a dragon in the ocean and sky,
Or as a cloud swirling around the moon.
The images of this art are without beginning or end.
You balance, intoxicated, on a leaping dragon fish.

The original calligraphy of this poem is reproduced on page 72. The lines were composed by Grand Master Wang Xiang Zhai. The scroll was commissioned and presented to me in Beijing by his daughter and spiritual heir, Madame Wang Yuk Fong. As the additional calligraphy on the scroll indicates, this gift conferred on me the responsibility for continuing Grand Master Wang Xiang Zhai's art.

In the lines of the poem, Grand Master Wang describes the inner experience of his art. He begins with the internal sensations of practicing Zhan Zhuang. The muscles, habitually tense and giving us the sensation of solidity, are deeply relaxed – as if the entire body structure was held from above by a puppet master. Our spirit is not dulled, however; on the contrary, our nervous system is fully alert – the hairs on our skin are keenly sensitive even to the slightest movement of the air around us. The mind, clear and still, is wide open: it is "seeing the three thousand" – a classical Chinese phrase meaning all phenomena, everything and everyone.

Internally, we are extraordinarily sensitive to the most subtle movements and changes within our organs and tissues.

The final four lines of the poem are devoted to the experience of movement in Da Cheng Chuan. First, the dragon: this mythical being has always been a symbol of immense wisdom and power. Dragons have the ability to inhabit all regions, from the celestial clouds to the depths of the earth and the seas. Their powerful bodies, sheathed in thousands of scales moving rhythmically and harmoniously in waves, are endowed with mysterious flexibility. Thus, in Da Cheng Chuan, unlike many other martial arts, there are no fixed routines and no repetitive "forms." Motion and stillness are its only forms, taking their constantly changing shapes from the energetic power of the practitioner, like "a cloud swirling around the moon."

Grand Master Wang found inspiration for Da Cheng Chuan from many different art forms – including poetry, painting, calligraphy and music – as well as from China's great philosophies and from his own careful observation of nature. The endless display of energy in all life provided him with images "without beginning or end" with which he described the essence of his art.

The combined sensitivity and strength that you develop through the practice of Da Cheng Chuan produce a feeling of being completely exhilarated, yet perfectly balanced. This is the experience Grand Master Wang expresses in the final line of his poem – being intoxicated with an abundance of energy, able to balance on the twisting scales of "a leaping dragon fish."

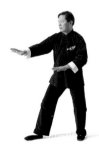

Tortoise in the Sea *Flick through the following pages (ending at page 99) to see Master Lam practice the Shih Li movement – Tortoise in the Sea (pages 138–139).* **1**

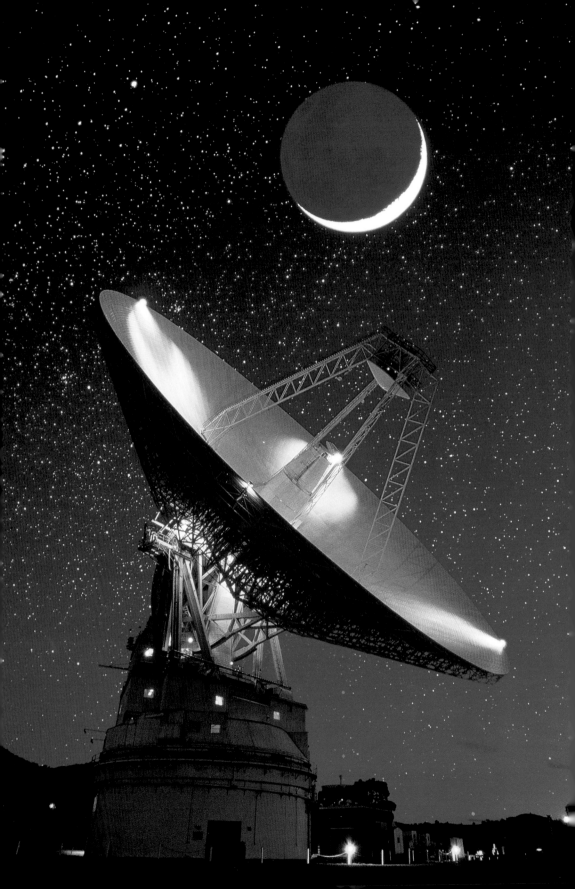

The Way

When we gaze at the night sky we feel the immense power of the universe. When we practice Zhan Zhuang we experience its primordial energy. This feeling, almost inexpressible, was conveyed by the great sage Lao Tse when he wrote:

> *It existed, like a mystery,*
> *Born before Heaven and Earth,*
> *Silent, limitless,*
> *Standing alone and unchanging –*
> *Present everywhere.*
> *We call it the mother of the ten thousand things.*
> *I do not know its name.*
> *Let us call it, "The Way."*

When we stand in the Zhan Zhuang postures, the natural curves of our arms and legs and the relaxed state of our body open us up to the energy of the cosmos. Like the receptor dish of a radio telescope, we attract and receive signals.

You cannot think your way into this experience. You have to feel it. Your heart is the key. Open your spirit outwards like the central receptor of a telescope, beckoning and welcoming the galaxies.

When we stand upright, with our hearts open, we are aerials, poised erect between the energy of the earth and the energy of space. Our feet take in earth energy through the sensitive points of our soles and, by being relaxed, we attract the magnetic energy of the universe to our head and body.

There is another "reception point" in the middle of the lower back – the acupuncture point known as Ming Men, the Gate of Life (page 20). If you do your Zhan Zhuang training outdoors, try standing so that the sun's rays fall on your back. Your Ming Men will naturally connect with that solar power.

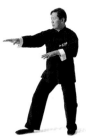

2

Your Energy

The energy of a tree is constantly flowing. It carries nutrition up from the roots to the leaves. Sugar, created from sunlight, water and carbon dioxide, moves down, feeding cells and promoting outward expansion. If you place a stethoscope against a cherry tree, or any other tree with smooth bark, you can hear it gurgling inside, especially in spring.

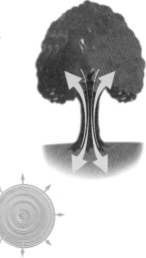

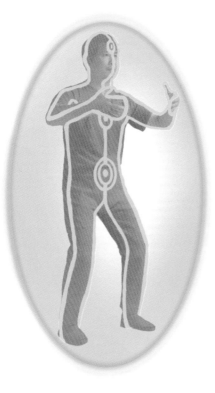

Within the body, the main reservoir of Chi energy is the Tan Tien in the lower abdomen. It circulates upwards to the middle Tan Tien in the center of the chest and the upper Tan Tien, often called "The Third Eye." Chi goes to the top of the head and then down to the feet, branching out to the hands, and returns again to the belly. It also flows around your entire body as your aura. Seen from above, your aura is centered over the top of your head.

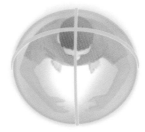

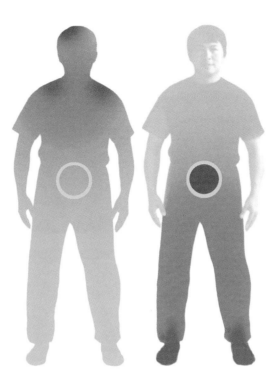

Stress can block energy in the upper body (left); Zhan Zhuang fills your Tan Tien and stabilizes your Chi (right).

Chi is something that we cannot see, touch or hear. But we can sense it and see its effects. For example, we cannot see the wind, but we can feel it and see its results. Sometimes, we use the word Chi to mean breath or gas. Chi is actually a wide variety of things ranging from gas to our aura, from a sensation that you feel to an impression that is made by a person even before you see them.

Zhan Zhuang not only strengthens your Chi, it readjusts its flow in your body. Many people suffer from blockages which trap most of their Chi in their upper body. They have headaches, stiff shoulders and tight chests. Since there is insufficient Chi in their lower body, they have digestive disorders, weak circulation in the legs and poor balance. When you practice Zhan Zhuang, your head is clearer and your upper body relaxed. The Chi reservoir in your lower Tan Tien is full and you are stable on your feet.

3

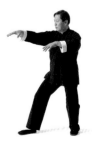

Human Architecture

Human architecture is based on a series of circles and triangles. These have the strength to carry considerable weight, yet keep your body flexible. You can think of your entire body as a pyramid, with a solid base and a much smaller apex. The three circles represent your head, torso and lower body. The tiny circles represent your neck and waist, supporting the structure while giving you the flexibility around which the larger spheres turn and roll.

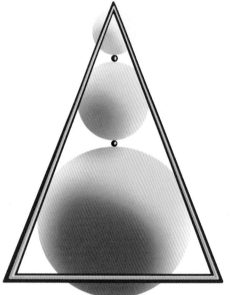

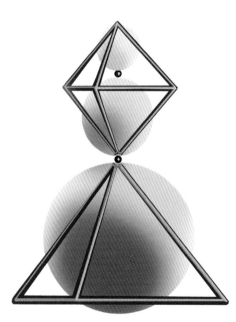

Within the principal pyramid structure, your body takes the shape of three smaller pyramids stacked one above the other. As they descend, they are progressively heavier. The mechanical principle of the neck and waist can be clearly seen in this structural model: a spherical pivot, like a ball bearing, bears the weight of the larger spheres and the convergence of the pyramids. Zhan Zhuang trains you in the proper alignment of these structures.

This model shows not only your physical structure, but also the principal lines of your energetic geometry. It includes the physical connections between the shoulders, elbows, hips and knees, as well as the relations between your three major Tan Tien energy centers.

The dotted lines at the top and bottom of the model indicate the opposing polarities of the energetic pulls experienced when you practice Zhan Zhuang. The white balloon between the knees is a reminder of the slight exertion you use to keep your knees properly aligned when standing in the postures.

A long loop from the shoulders goes down around the lower Tan Tien. This indicates the energetic stability of the whole structure. Your Chi is centered in your lower abdomen. This abdominal center of gravity is shown in popular dolls, known as Bei Tao Yung, literally "the old people who never fall down."

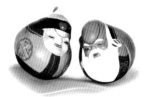

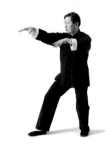

4

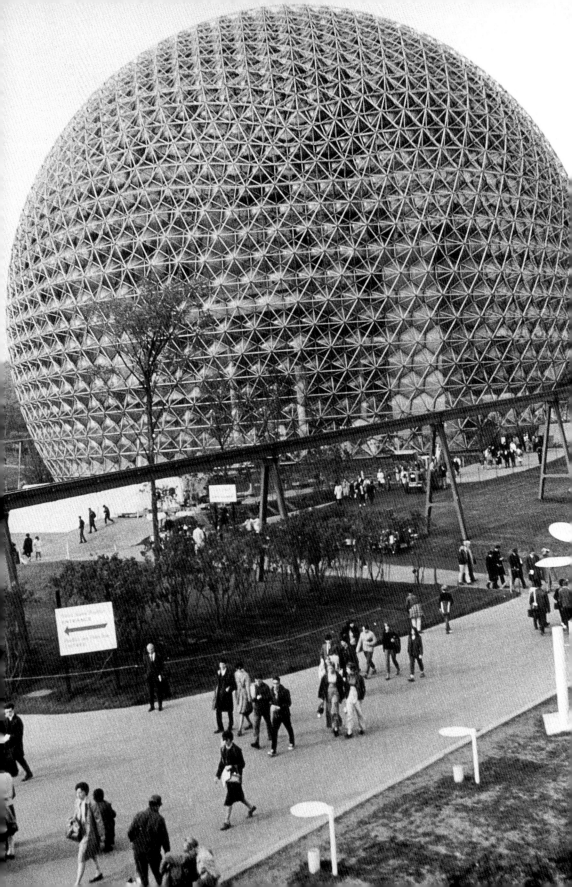

The Web

Contemporary science has revealed that underlying patterns of energy are entirely in accord with the earliest wisdom of Chinese naturalists who studied the subtle workings of the human body.

One of the most striking examples of structural energy is the geodesic dome. One of the best known is the 80 m (250 ft)-high sphere on the left, constructed for an international exposition in Montreal. The largest is about 23 times the volume of the dome on St. Peter's Basilica in Rome.

The dome's strength comes from a web of triangles and circles, two of nature's most resilient structures. The "omnitriangulated" dome is completely stable, yet flexible. In an early experiment, a dome made of 170 aluminium struts, weighing only 30 kg (65 lb) was able to support a total load of six tons – the equivalent of a canoe bearing the weight of an army tank.

The triangles and curves disperse tension outwards the way gas evenly expands the rubber skin of a balloon. In fact, the dome's compression struts can maintain the web of support even if they are not all physically touching. The pattern itself acts as an "energetic network" sustaining a firm structural pattern. Some physicists have concluded that these innovative structures may, in fact, be models of an atom's nuclear structure.

It is the same principle that enables a spider's web to float intact in hurricane force winds.

Some domes have been called "gossamer nets" while others have been described as "a single, finite, energetic embrace." The genius who invented the geodesic dome, Buckminster Fuller, said the structure performed according to the theories of Energetic Geometry, following the laws of the cosmos. He called these energetic patterns "the personal, regenerative energy" through which the universe works.

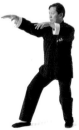

5

The Pump

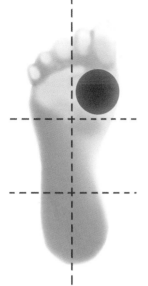

Your training teaches you how to move and control the flow of Chi through the energetic geometry of your body. The first stage is to ensure the correct alignment of your body and to clear any obstacles you may have to the free flow of energy through your system. This is what you accomplish by the practice of Zhan Zhuang. When you have become stable in that practice, which also results in an overall increase in your energy levels, the focus of your training moves to your feet. Imagine the sole of your foot is divided into six sections. Focus your attention on the section shown here with a red ball.

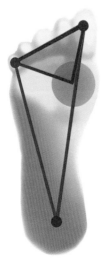

When you stand in the Zhan Zhuang postures, experiment with the difference between standing on the full triangle of your foot and the much smaller red triangle. When you stand with your weight evenly spread across your full foot, you emphasize the health aspect of your training. The work you do with pressure on the red triangle unlocks the secrets of the explosive power of Da Cheng Chuan.

You can see the same architecture in your
foot when looking at it from the side. One
triangle is formed by the ankle, big toe
and heel. A second triangle is formed by
the ankle, ball of the foot and heel. A third
triangle is formed by the ankle, big toe and
ball of the foot. For the martial aspect of Da
Cheng Chuan, you need to understand and
use the power of this third triangle.

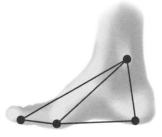

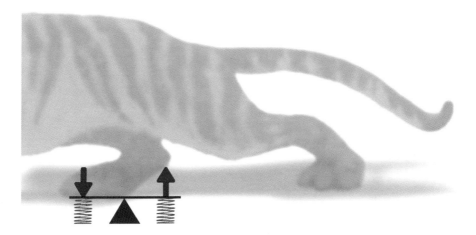

The soles of your feet have a remarkable structure that enables
them to bear weight, yet remain sensitive and spring-like. The
arch of your foot acts like a fulcrum. When pressure is applied
downwards onto the ball of the foot, a corresponding upward
spring of the heel carries on through the ankle and upwards
through the structure of your body. This same principle is used
to develop and pump your Chi for use in the advanced stages
of Da Cheng Chuan.

6

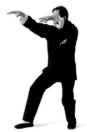

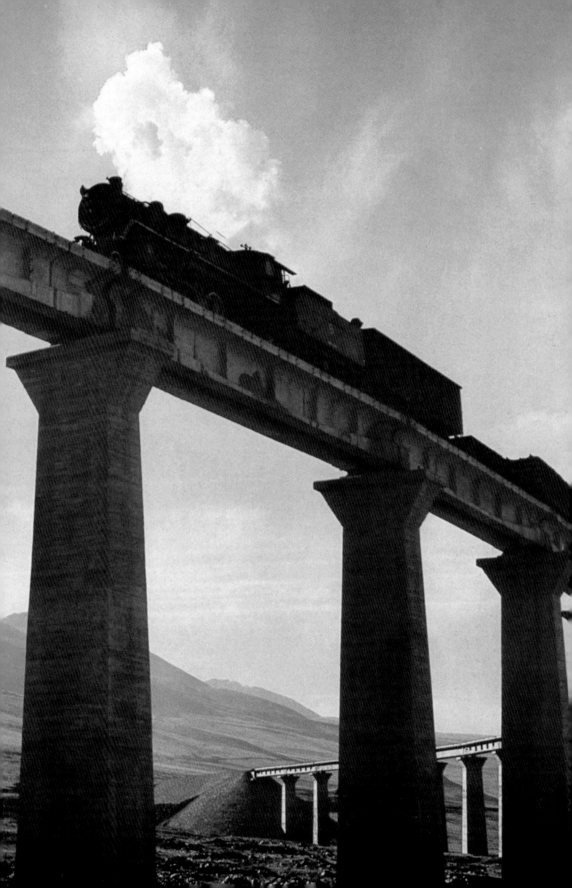

The Bridge

If you look carefully at the point where the pillars of a bridge bear the structure's enormous weight, you will often find a small cylinder. This astonishing feature is known as a "bridge bearing." The purpose of the bearing is to take the weight while giving the entire structure maximum flexibility.

Bridge bearings transfer loads and movements from the deck of the bridge down to the substructure and foundations. They make it possible for the structure to withstand the vibrations of traffic and the expansion and contraction caused by temperature variations. It is also thanks to these bearings that bridges are able to withstand severe winds, tremors and earthquakes.

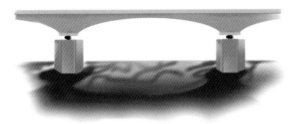

The bearings are designed to redirect the forces that move over, through and around the structure. Engineers study the "downward forces" that pass through the center of the bearing, the "transverse forces" that move horizontally through the bridge or alongside it, the "uplift forces" that enter the structure from the earth and "rotational forces" that can twist in any direction.

Our feet have a natural bridge-like structure, arching between the ball and heel. They, too, have the capacity to absorb and redirect forces moving in all directions. Training to use the "red triangle" (pages 84–85) takes advantage of this natural structure and greatly increases your ability to react to and redirect forces all around you.

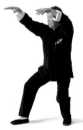

7

Power Training

To begin this stage of your training, stand in Wu Chi for five minutes with your weight spread evenly over your feet. Then, shift your weight slightly forwards. Let your heels come up just enough to slide a sheet of paper under them. Focus your weight: it should rest on the red triangle shown on page 84. Include this new development in your daily training, so that you are able to remain balanced and stable without any weight on your heels. Progress to the point where you can maintain all the Zhan Zhuang postures, including those on one leg, using only the "red triangles" of your feet.

As you stand in this advanced position, you will naturally engage your large calf muscles. The next stage of this practice is to focus your attention on those muscles, particularly the large gastrocnemius muscle in the bulge of your calf. Try to identify it so that you are able to contract it for several seconds without engaging the muscles of your ankle, thigh or buttock and while keeping your upper body completely relaxed.

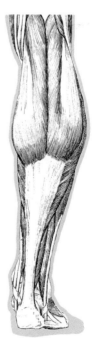

Once you have trained your nerves to contract and relax the muscles in both calves, include this in your daily training. Contract and relax the muscles in your left calf up to 30 times, then do the same for your right calf. Then try contracting and relaxing both calves together. Avoid tensing any other muscles: focus your training on the nerves that control the muscles of your calves.

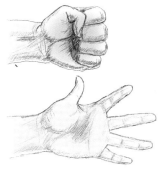

This training develops your internal sensitivity, exercises your nerves and sharpens the ability of your central nervous system to control subtle movements within your body. There is a similar practice for your hands. When you stand in the Zhan Zhuang posture, Holding the Ball (page 13), tighten your left hand into a fist. Squeeze it tightly for about five seconds. Then release the fist and open your hand fully. Stretch your fingers as wide apart as possible. Hold for about five seconds. Then repeat up to 30 times. Do the same with your other hand. When you practice closing and opening each hand, pay particular attention to your upper arms, shoulders and chest: these should remain completely relaxed. If you notice muscles in your upper body tensing, direct your attention to them and relax them.

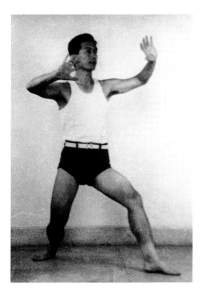

These two mind-training exercises can become part of your daily practice. Gradually increase the length of time you spend standing with your weight on the "red triangles" of your feet. To the untrained observer, your feet appear flat on the ground, but, as in this photograph of the young Professor Yu, you develop the pump that will transform your practice.

8

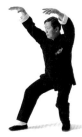

Deeper Strength

A deep connection with the earth is essential for your health and your martial arts power. You develop this connection through your Zhan Zhuang training and the advanced work on the "red triangle" of your foot (pages 84–89). To go further, you need to use the power of your imagination to draw more deeply on the energy of the earth. Clearly visualize the basic triangle from the tip of your head to the base of your feet. Imagine that your feet go straight down into the earth. As your practice deepens, you will feel a second, inverted triangle extending downwards and holding you to the earth.

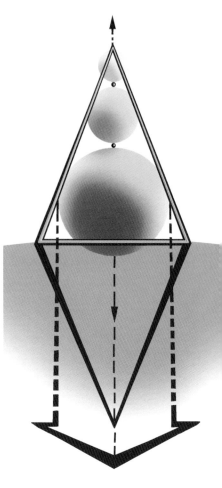

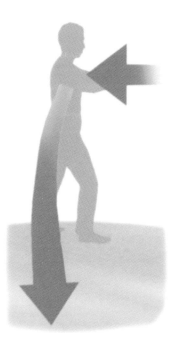

You can use this deep strength in the martial arts to take the incoming force of an attack into your body and direct it down through your rear leg. If you are learning for the first time, hold a Zhan Zhuang posture to one side and ask a friend to lean on your arms. Keep them in place without tension, directing the pressure down through your back foot.

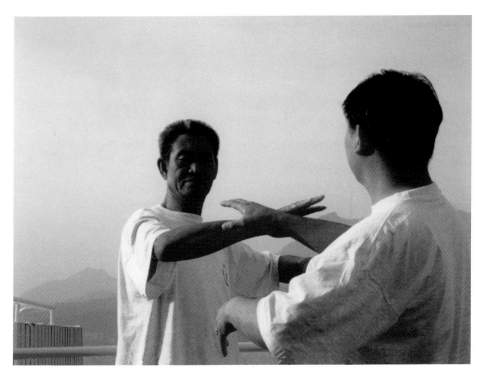

Through your Zhan Zhuang training, the energetic structure of
your body becomes increasingly stronger. Keeping this clearly in
mind is vital to the power of Da Cheng Chuan. It is the secret of
the relaxed strength of advanced practitioners, such as the two
masters in this photograph: facing Master Lam is Master Guo
Gui Zhi, three times national martial arts champion of China.

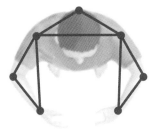

When the arms are held in the fundamental
Zhan Zhuang position, Holding the Ball
(page 13), three principal triangles are
involved. Two are formed by the shoulder,
elbow and wrist of each arm. The third runs
from shoulder to shoulder and connects to
the first thoracic vertebra of the spine. These
three triangles, combining structural and
energetic geometry, remain intact under all
pressures, but move flexibly without tension.

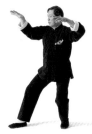

9

Building Pressure

We can think of Chi as pressure. The classical ideogram of Chi has two parts. On top is a square that represents a container or pot with a handle. Below that are four strokes that symbolize fire. So the whole character represents the process of heating something over a fire. It is a process of transforming something by energizing it. For example, it could be water, which when boiled, produces steam.

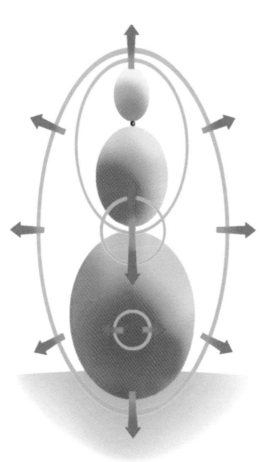

We are completely familiar with the pressure of steam. We are also familiar with the pressure of Chi. This is the power that moves our blood, fuels the extraordinary complexity of our entire nervous system, gives vitality to our internal organs and stimulates our brain cells. If we increase the power of our Chi, we increase its pressure. This boosts the energy circulating throughout our entire system. The energy radiates outwards from the Tan Tien in the lower abdomen, passes through every region of the body and extends beyond us.

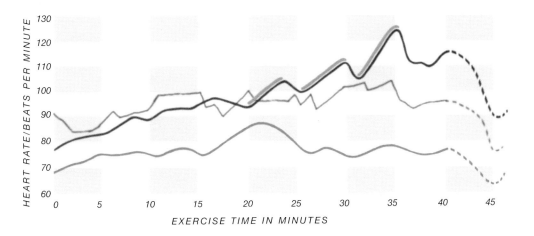

The power exercises you are learning increase the pressure exerted by your Chi, boosting your circulation and bathing all your cells in oxygen-rich blood. This chart shows the impact on different people, measured in terms of pulse rates.

Blue line. An anxious patient begins with a pulse of 91 beats per minute. His pulse lowers slightly as he relaxes in Wu Chi. He is guided through Zhan Zhuang positions that progressively stimulate his circulation and deepen his breathing. Five minutes after the session, his pulse is at a much healthier 76 a minute.

Green line. A long-term student undertakes 40 minutes of demanding practice, holding eight of the postures in this book. As a result of sustained Zhan Zhuang training, her pulse remains smooth, slow and powerful throughout.

Red line. This advanced practitioner demonstrates the power of "red triangle" training. He remains completely still, but his pulse rate escalates dramatically (shown in orange) when he uses the power training technique explained on pages 88–89. This same explosive energy, known as Fa Li or Fa Jing, can be released in a split second by accomplished Da Cheng Chuan practitioners.

10

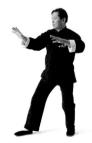

Power Circles

The strength you develop in your training begins to express itself throughout your entire body. Not only do you experience an unshakable connection to the earth, but if you bump into something or someone hits you, the impact just seems to bounce naturally off you.

In this model, the outer sphere represents your muscle. Its structure is like a powerful rubber ball: it can support heavy weights, but also compress to accept pressure. The triangle is bone. Its structure is like that of a bamboo: it provides strong structural support and keeps the outer circle of muscle firmly balanced. Inside the bone is your Chi, represented by the inner glowing sphere. This is the deep energy developed by your Zhan Zhuang practice: it moves within the marrow of your bones.

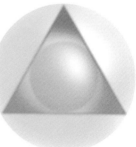

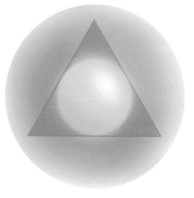

The energy within the bone marrow, like all energy, radiates naturally outwards in all directions. This is happening all the time, but bursts of radiating energy can be triggered by the power of the Tan Tien in your lower abdomen.

When your Chi expands outwards from the bone marrow, it presses on the entire structure of the bone. That power extends out into the muscle, which spontaneously expands like an air cushion.

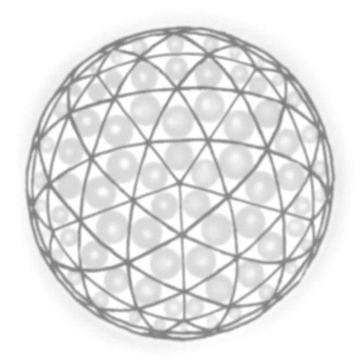

The diagrams on the facing page show the workings of energy in a single sliver of the body. You can imagine the effect of your Chi power multiplied millions of times throughout your entire body. As each circle of energy expands outwards, it immediately comes into contact with the other radiating spheres around it. The effect is like the vast chain reaction in nuclear fission.

This is exactly the process that happens inside your body as a result of advanced Da Cheng Chuan training. Your Tan Tien acts as the center of a vast web of circles and triangles. Directed by your mental power, your Chi can be trained to expand rapidly outwards, setting off a similar reaction throughout the millions of power centers in your system. At this stage, your power can be released from any single point on your body. At the higher stages, your entire aura itself can become a field of power.

11

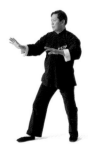

Breaking Through

Grand Master Wang Xiang Zhai is famous for telling his disciples: "A large movement is not as good as a small movement. A small movement is not as good as no movement at all." Since he was training them in combat, it was hard to comprehend this at first. Then they came to realize through their practice that no matter how fast you move your muscles and perform an external movement, it is not as fast as an internal movement of energy. Once you have trained the whole body to move and react as a single unit, even the smallest adjustment of your position becomes a powerful expression of the energy of the whole body.

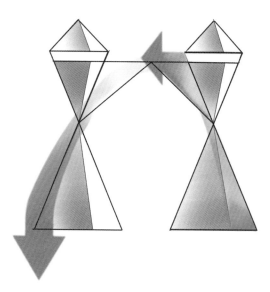

You can understand this principle by seeing how the structural and energetic geometry of the body, combined with the inner workings of your Chi, enables your entire energy field to react to an external stimulus. In this simplified model, the incoming impact from an opponent is immediately absorbed through the relaxed musculature of the body and instantly transmitted down into the earth. There is a corresponding, natural reaction which transmits amplified energy back towards the opponent. You appear motionless, but your opponent bounces off helplessly as the energy response does its work.

You can think of this energy response as the action of a catapult that is fully drawn and about to release a stone. It is also similar to a bow about to release an arrow. Your energy is in a perpetual state of readiness, capable of being released at any moment. This is the practical meaning of the words of Grand Master Wang Xiang Zhai, when he told his students: "Preserve your strength like a bow that has been fully drawn."

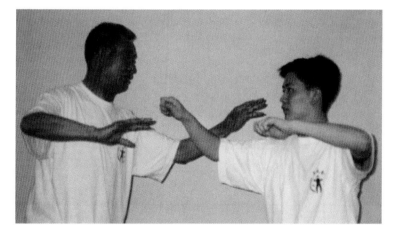

Master Guo Yi Zhi practices the Da Cheng Chuan energy exchange through single hand contact with Lam Tin Hun who has studied the art under his father, Master Lam Kam Chuen.

Initially, your experience of this spontaneous energy response may be more like that of a hard rubber ball. If you throw it against a wall, it changes shape slightly to take the impact. But the natural reaction of the rubber snaps it back into shape and it rebounds with greater force.

12

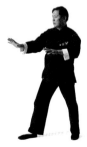

Your Natural Strength: Protection

Your field of energy gives you protection. It helps to prevent accidents, can be used in emergencies and will help you recover if you are injured.

As you deepen your practice of Da Cheng Chuan, the energy surrounding you becomes stronger and extends further out from your body. It acts like a natural radar system. You become aware of possible dangers far earlier and further away from you than you did before. Your field of vision is broader and your mind becomes aware of obstacles before they are in full view.

Your training strengthens your nervous system. When you are put to a sudden test, you are more patient, calm and able to think clearly. You tire less and feel more resilient.

As you develop the five powers that are explained in Part Four and the stepping movements shown in Part Five, you discover a natural coordination that subconsciously protects you. Students who have had potentially dangerous accidents on dark streets, been attacked or fallen, find they remain in balance. They move easily out of the way with intuitive speed or spontaneously use their hands and feet to break their fall without serious injury.

If you have an accident or injury, you can draw on your Zhan Zhuang training for emergency help. If you are knocked down, fall or are hit, the first principle is to remain still immediately afterwards. You should only move if you are in actual danger. For example, if you are knocked off your bicycle and are not severely hurt, move to a safe spot nearby and then remain still. Any severe shock will automatically disturb your entire energy system. However, your energy naturally seeks to rebalance itself and will do this very rapidly so long as the entire body remains still. If it is at all possible, try to lie, sit or stand in a Zhan Zhuang posture. Then, before moving or while being transported, practice Sealing your Energy (page 15).

Your training gives you inner resources of Chi. Like this ancient statue carved in the rocks of Yungang – an area of China where Da Cheng Chuan is regarded as "the training of a Buddha" – your power envelops you like a protective mountain.

If you are injured and conscious, warm your hands (either by rubbing them or clapping them together) and then hold your injury if you can. You can wrap your hands around most twisted joints and broken bones or place them over an open wound. Your Chi will warm and protect the injured area, speeding the flow of healing energy. It will also help reduce blood loss. You can do this for yourself but you can also use your healing power in the same way to calm and assist others.

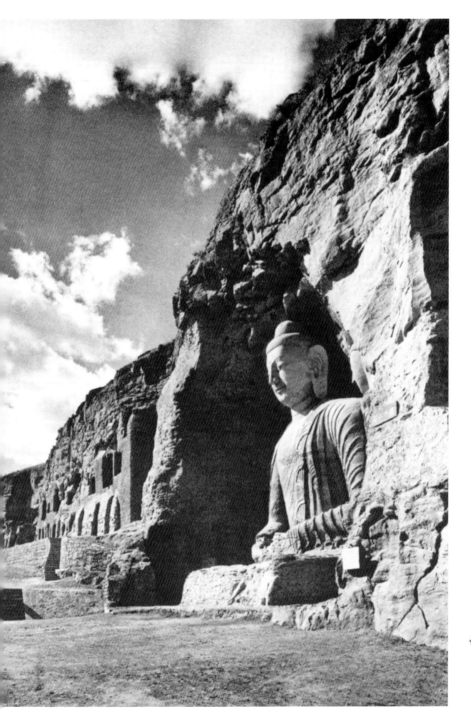

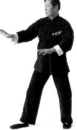

13

THE GREAT ACCOMPLISHMENT LINEAGE III

As he journeyed from master to master, learning and studying their martial techniques, Grand Master Wang Xiang Zhai increasingly focused his attention on the inner essence of their art. This was more important than the superficial differences between styles. For him the great accomplishment of the martial arts did not lie in the repetition of classical "forms" consisting of set movements. Real power lay in the cultivation of the internal energy that could be directed by the mind.

By the time he began teaching publicly in Shanghai in the 1920s, he had distilled his learning into a system that placed mental power first. He called his system Yi Chuan, literally "Mind Fist," often translated as "Intention Boxing."

When he began teaching in Beijing in the 1940s, his system was acclaimed as The Great Accomplishment – Da Cheng Chuan. Eminent martial artists from China and Japan tried their techniques on him, but found themselves effortlessly bounced off by his power. Respectfully, they asked to become his students. Even earlier in Shanghai, a European world boxing champion had tried to knock out the diminutive master with a single punch and was floored. He was so startled, he reported it to *The Times* newspaper in London.

Grand Master Wang broke new ground by challenging the traditional secrecy of martial arts instruction. He taught openly.

"Knowledge should not be hidden away like a secret," he declared, "it belongs to all humanity."

In 1993, on the 30th anniversary of his death, Grand Master Wang's long-term disciples in China (many of them in their 80s and 90s) and a delegation of recent Zhan Zhuang students from countries around the world gathered for a commemorative ceremony in Beijing. The events took place at his tomb (page 154) and included a seminar at the World Health Organization Collaborating Center for Occupational Health.

Many of Grand Master Wang's disciples are pictured on the facing page, grouped around his daughter Madame Wang Yuk Fong. In a talk to Western students, Madame Wang told them to be attentive while holding the Zhan Zhuang posture, but to smile at the same time. "This is the 'inner laughter,'" she said. "That inner happiness will continue through your whole life. The more you stand, the more comfortable you feel. Everything looks very soft, relaxed and at ease. Yet there is immense power inside you."

"If you study and practice Zhan Zhuang you can easily live to over a hundred!" said Master Li Jian Yu, Chief of the International Education Department of the Beijing Wushu Association. "Just stand quietly, listening to the sounds of the birds and noticing the internal movements of energy in your body. This is the pathway to a long life!"

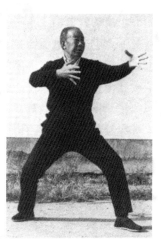
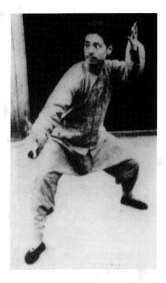
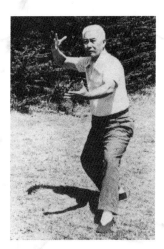
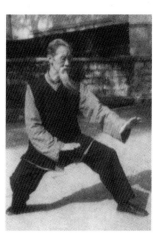
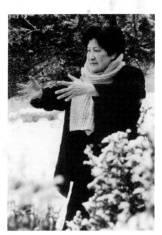
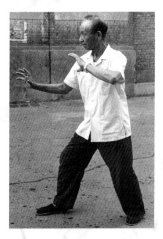
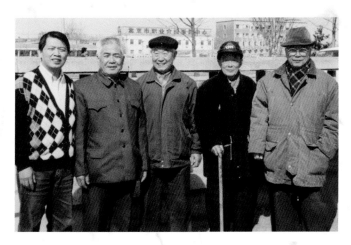
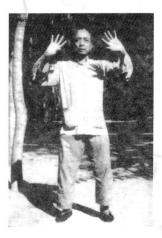

將相胸懷儒學問

英雄肝膽佛心腸

THE FORCES OF NATURE

Calligraphy of twin couplets, described in the Introduction to Part Four.

The heart of a general,
The mind of Confucius

The bravery of a hero,
The compassion of a Buddha.

The original calligraphy of these twin couplets is reproduced
on the opening page of Part Four (page 102). The two scrolls
were composed and hand drawn as a gift to me by one of the
personal bodyguards of Dr. Sun Yat Sen, the founder of modern
China who became the country's first president.

The couplets offer heart advice for anyone contemplating the
martial arts. In many places today the martial arts tradition has
been misunderstood and reduced merely to a collection of
punches and combat movements. Of course, the invincibility of
an accomplished martial artist is well known. But that power
does not come from aggressive techniques. The source of true
power is found in these lines from Dr. Sun Yat Sen's bodyguard.

The "heart of a general" refers to the qualities of a good leader:
open-mindedness, generosity and the ability to work with,
understand and motivate people. "The mind of Confucius"
signifies deep learning, wisdom and knowledge. The meaning
of this line is not restricted to that one philosopher, but to all who
have devoted themselves to the path of profound understanding.
"The bravery of a hero" is born of fearlessness, the essence of
human freedom. "The compassion of a Buddha" blossoms from
an open heart and a mind as vast as the universe itself.

Understanding these four qualities is particularly important at this
stage in your training since Part Four introduces you to the martial application of your power. You will be learning and practicing

the five power movements from the Da Cheng Chuan tradition. But it would be a serious mistake to think that what you will learn is how to be violent. "With profound knowledge," wrote Grand Master Wang Xiang Zhai, "this helps to mold your temperament, cultivating you in faithfulness, sense of justice, benevolence and bravery." The whole point of this practice, he declared, was not victory or defeat, but to achieve "comfort, increase your strength and put zest into your life."

When teaching his disciples, Grand Master Wang said that his art could not be understood only through scientific explanation. He stressed that it must be intuitively grasped through direct practice. "What can be explained are the mechanics of strength; the inexplicable lies within your mind," he said.

Those who admired Grand Master Wang called his system The Great Accomplishment because instead of teaching them a fixed set of movements, he communicated the essence of the human power that was being expressed. This gave his students great freedom, enabling them to move with new strength without being constrained by the repetitive imitation of dead forms.

The five movements described on pages 108 to 127 reflect the traditional Chinese system of the Five Energies. These are the five principal directions in which energy moves. The Five Energies are said to direct all natural cycles such as the seasons and to express themselves in the forces of nature. It was these forces that Grand Master Wang Xiang Zhai learned to unleash in the art of Da Cheng Chuan.

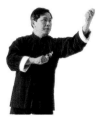

Water Power *Flick through the following pages with your thumb (ending at page 129) to see Master Lam demonstrate the arm movements that express Water Power (pages 112–115).* **1**

Full Swing

For the five Da Cheng Chuan movements in this part of the book, you need to work at releasing any residual tension stored in your joints. This is essential because it is such tension that will constrict the full movement and block the flow of energy. This exercise concentrates on freeing up your shoulders and hips.

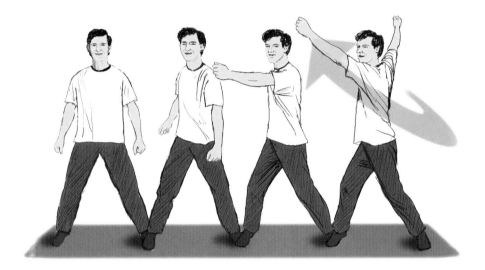

Start with your feet shoulder width apart. Settle down and do your best to relax your shoulders, chest, back and hips. If you are feeling a little tense, first do the three preliminary exercises that loosen your shoulders, hips and knees. These are explained in Part One (pages 20–25): Opening the Inner Gate, Arm Circles and Knees Up.

Turn your hips to the right. Your left heel will naturally rise a little off the ground. As you turn, fling both your arms upwards. Then turn back to the center, letting your arms come down and turn your hips to the left, flinging your arms upwards as you turn.

In the beginning, this motion may seem a little stiff. You might experience difficulty in getting your arms fully extended above your head. You may find you can turn only a little to either side. In that case, spend more time working with the three preliminary exercises and perform this full swing very gently.

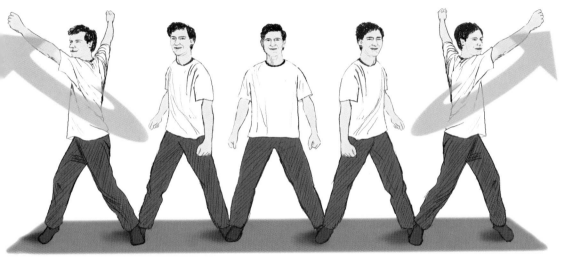

As your practice develops, you should aim to turn your hips and torso like a stallion rearing its head around to the side so that you send your arms speeding upwards like the flying hairs on the horse's mane.

Start with 10 complete swings to each side, if you can. Then work towards 30 to each side.

2

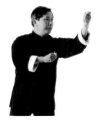

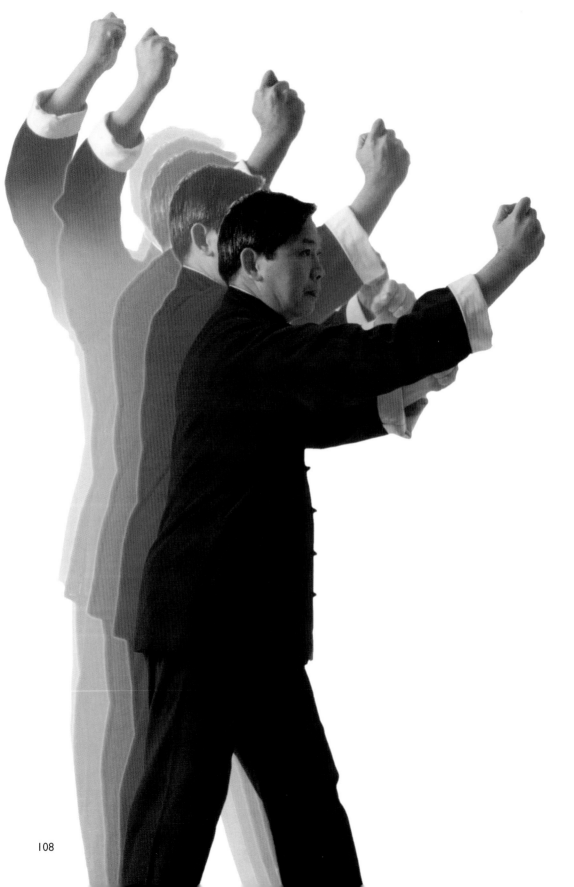

Metal

Begin this practice in Wu Chi. Release any tension in your neck, shoulders, chest and hips. Then slowly raise your arms into the position, Holding the Ball (page 13). Your previous training in this position is important to ensure that the full weight of your arms is resting completely on the imaginary balloons under your armpits, upper arm and forearm.

Fold your hands into loose fists. Do not clench them. Connect the pads of your thumbs to the first knuckle of your forefingers. This creates an arrowhead on each fist.

Raise both arms up beside the right side of your head, your right fist held higher than your left. Slice down to the left, bringing both fists to the level of your chest, your lower fist stopping opposite the center of your torso.

Then raise both arms up beside the left side of your head, with your left fist held higher than your right. Slice down to the right, again bringing both fists to the level of your chest. Your lower fist stops opposite the center of your torso.

Feel as if you are holding a large axe in your hands and then strike powerful blows from one side to the other. Maintain the alignment of your fists at the end of each blow, so that the full force of the blow is expressed by your forearms.

Once you become familiar with the chopping motion, change the position of your feet: turn one foot 45 degrees outwards and step forwards with the other. Look straight ahead as you continue chopping.

Begin gradually, paying attention to the correct movement of your arms. The action should be smooth, light and relaxed. Start slowly. Build up to 30 times. When you can do the movement without tensing, practice as many as you wish.

3

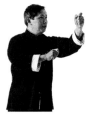

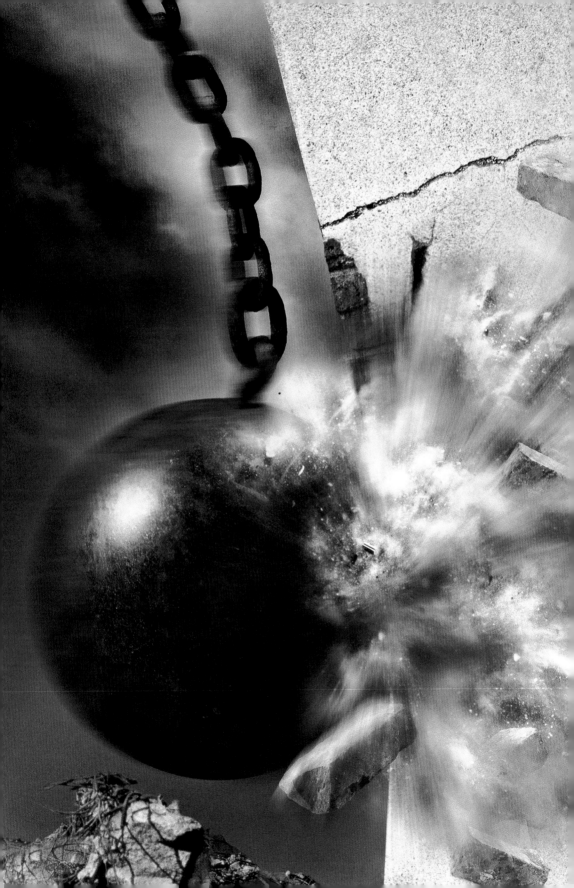

Metal Power

The power that is expressed through the Metal punch is one of the primal forces known in Chinese as the Five Energies. Metal energy is highly condensed, giving it enduring strength. In nature, metal makes its appearance deep within the earth. It has the power to cut almost all other known materials. When sharpened, like the blade of a sword or the head of an axe, it is lethal.

Metal Power is greater than that of the physical metal. In the words of Grand Master Wang Xiang Zhai: "Metal is the power contained in the bones and muscles, the mind being firm like iron or stone, able to cut gold or steel."

As you train in this movement, imagine you are wielding a heavy axe into thick timber. The axe head sinks into the wood. You feel a corresponding shudder through your body as the momentum of your energy rebounds from the blow. Working with this image establishes the cutting power in your mind.

The full expression of Metal goes deeper still. In your mind you experience the immense weight of a single blow smashing completely through whatever stands in front of you – a huge block of timber, a steel post, a stone column, a mountain. As you train with these images in your mind, you unleash the power of an iron wrecking ball levelling an entire building.

This power is not only physical, nor is it limited to the martial arts. Each of the Five Energies expresses itself along a spectrum that includes the physical, emotional, mental and spiritual. These energies take coarse and subtle forms. Cultivating your Metal energy hones your mental clarity. It gives you the power to cut through confusion, to get straight to the point. You learn to communicate with precision and express the truth without fear.

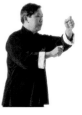

4

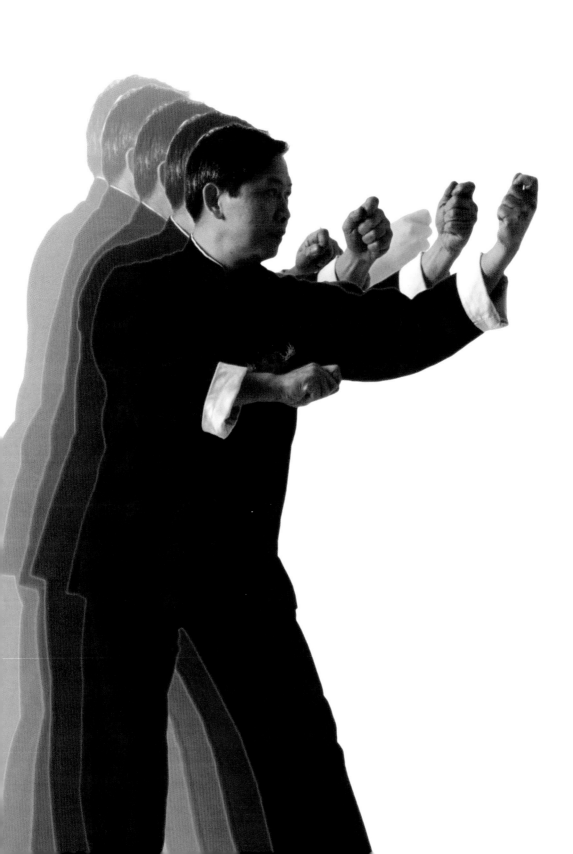

Water 水

Begin in Wu Chi. Then slowly raise your arms into the position, Holding the Ball (page 13). Ensure the full weight of your arms rests completely on the imaginary balloons under them.

Fold your hands into loose fists, with the pads of your thumbs contacting the first knuckle of your forefingers. This creates a arrowhead on each fist.

Twist one fist while raising it in front of you until your arm is directed 45 degrees away from your body. Your extended fist is opposite the center of your forehead.

Bring your arm back down to chest level, unwinding the twist. Your hand rests close to the center of your chest. As you do this, make the upward twisting movement with the other hand.

Imagine you are holding a screwdriver and twisting its blade upwards and outwards in front of you. Make the fullest possible twist with each wrist, while doing your best to avoid tension in your chest and shoulders. Your eyes focus on the point in space where you direct the arrowhead of each fist.

Once you become familiar with the upward twisting arm motion, change the position of your feet: turn one foot 45 degrees outwards and step forwards with the other. Look straight ahead as you continue to twist your arms.

Begin gradually, paying attention to the correct movement of your arms. The action should be smooth, light and relaxed. Start slowly. Build up to 30 times. When you can do the movement with a flowing action that is free from tension, practice as many as you wish.

5

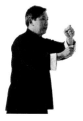

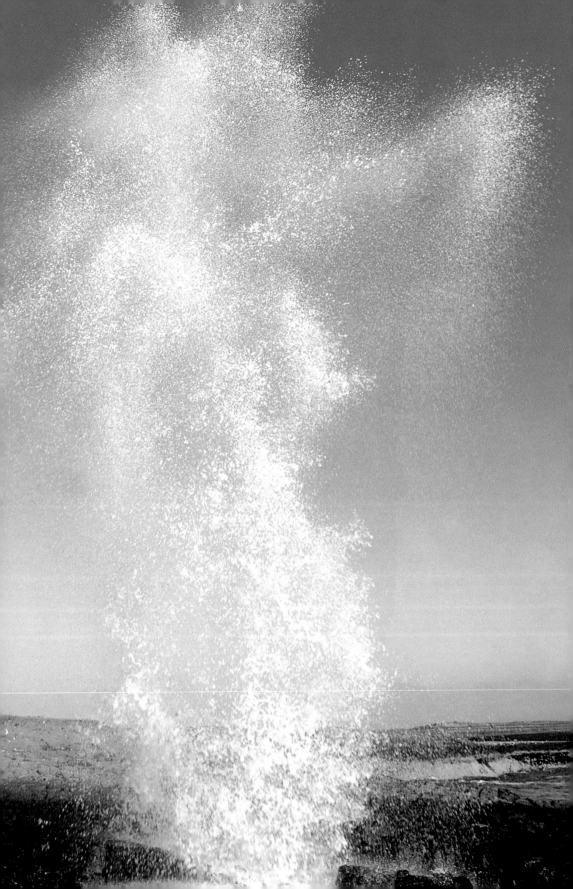

Water Power

Water Power is the second of the Five Energies. The nature of water makes it elusive, hard to grasp and impossible to resist. It takes many forms. As the ocean, it is vast, dangerous and deep. As the mist and rain, it moves formlessly, is all pervasive and takes the shape of whatever vessel it finds. As a waterfall, it crushes. As tiny droplets, it wears away stone. As a tornado or waterspout, it twists upwards with explosive power.

In the words of Grand Master Wang Xiang Zhai: "Water is a force like the waves of the vast sea; it is as lively as a dragon or snake. When used, it has the power to pervade everything."

The lively, dragon-like power of Water is forcefully expressed in this movement. You learn to twist your wrist as if stabbing upwards while turning a screwdriver in your hand. This trains you in the fundamental twisting motion.

The power of this movement is ungraspable, like a writhing snake. It is like an intense jet of water driving through a high-pressure hose. It is impossible to hold the hose completely still: it shakes and thunders in your hands.

The power which arises in your mind is of an upward rush of uncontrollable strength. It is like the force of a sandblaster or the sudden eruption of boiling steam.

As with all the Five Energies, Water Power manifests on many levels in human beings. This exercise gives you the strength to persist and to penetrate. It takes you to your target, overcoming the obstacles in your path, no matter how solid they may appear to be. This is the power to find different directions and solutions and to move swiftly when the moment is right.

6

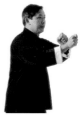

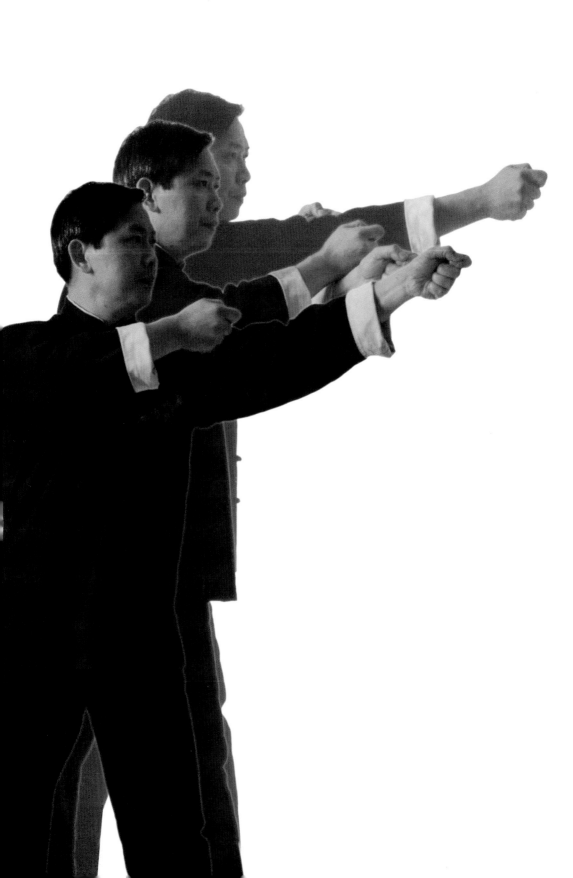

Wood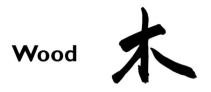

Begin in Wu Chi. Then slowly raise your arms into the position, Holding the Ball (page 13). Take the time to fully relax your chest and the muscles of your upper body.

Fold your hands into loose fists. Your fingertips are a hair's breadth away from your palms. Form an arrowhead on each fist by connecting the pads of your thumbs to the first knuckle of your forefingers.

Adjust the position of your hands so that they level with your chin and nose, one above the other. Do not bring them in too close to your face: always leave a little safety space.

Extend your topmost fist straight forwards, leading with the arrowhead. Then bring that fist back so that it comes under the other one. Then extend forwards with the fist that is now on top.

When you have mastered the correct motion of each arm, try making the movements simultaneously. Bring your extended fist back at the same time as you extend forwards with the other one. Pull your fist back with the same power as you drive forwards with the other.

Once you are familiar with the continuous forward movement, change the position of your feet: turn one foot 45 degrees outwards and step forwards with the other. Look straight ahead and continue extending your arms.

Start slowly. Build up to 30 times. When you are comfortable doing the continuous movement without tensing, practice for as long as you wish.

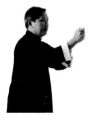

7

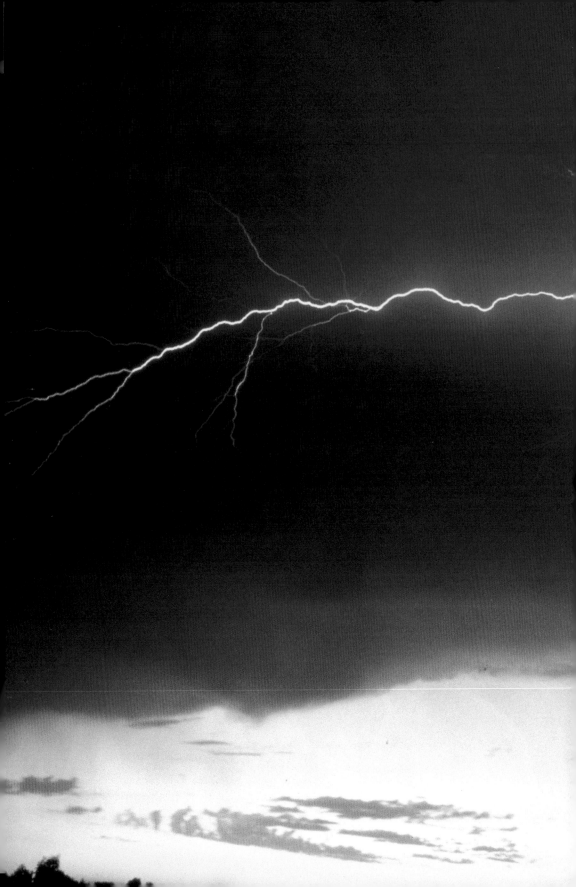

Wood Power

Wood Power is the third of the Five Energies. Traditionally, Wood energy is described as expanding, just as a tree grows outwards in all directions, year after year.

In the words of Grand Master Wang Xiang Zhai: "Wood is the yielding, yet rooted, power of a tree." This reminds us of the importance of the foundation practices (pages 11–15) that underlie all accomplishment in Da Cheng Chuan: without the deep rooting that develops from the standing practice of Zhan Zhuang, your body's external movements will be without power.

Wood Power draws its strength from the standing practice and then extends straight ahead. It has the force of lightning that streaks across the sky or an axe's blade shearing along a straight beam of timber.

You start to release blows like a volley of straight arrows, one after another in quick succession. Each cuts through the air, straight to its target.

Wood Power is greater than wood itself. It has the unstoppable, cutting speed of a chain saw. The chain is not stiff: your arm is never fully extended. The point of contact is as sharp as a drill: your fist is formed into an arrowhead.

The application of this power in the martial arts is renowned. It also influences the full spectrum of your energy field. Wood Power is resilient. It enables you to take an emotional or physical blow, absorb its impact and bounce back. You are not crushed by failure. Rather, like a tree, you can transform one form of energy into another. Like branches in the wind, you can return again and again. Fully concentrated, this power of the mind is like an archer.

8

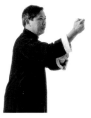

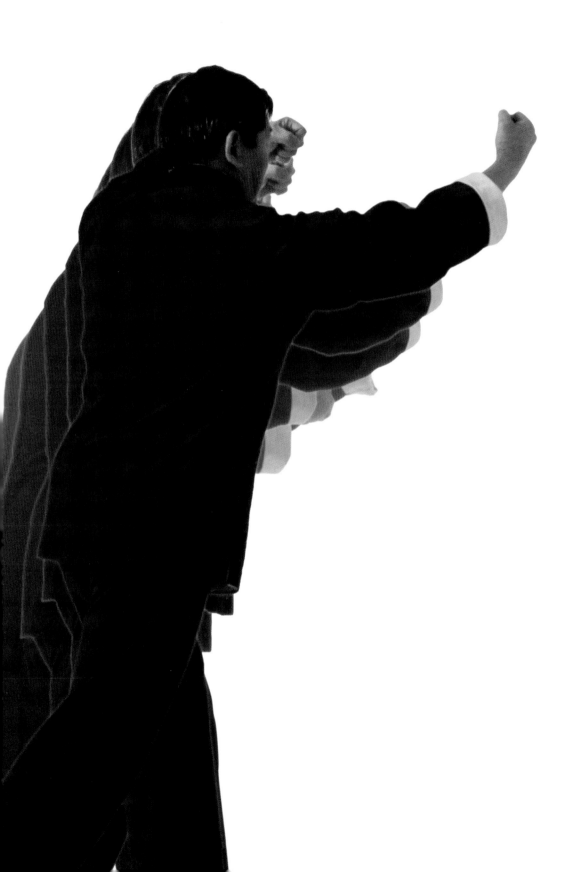

Fire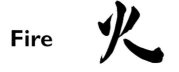

Begin your training in Wu Chi. Sink your weight fully into your feet and feel the light upward suspension at the top of your head. Then slowly raise your arms into the position, Holding the Ball (page 13). The complete relaxation of your shoulders and upper body is essential.

Make two loose fists, as if you were holding tiny eggs carefully in each hand. Do not clench your fingers. In each hand, connect the pad of your thumb to the first knuckle of your forefinger to make an arrowhead.

Start to the left. The motion begins in your hips. Turn them towards the left diagonal, keeping your feet firmly rooted to the ground. As your body turns to the left diagonal, raise your right arm in the direction of the turn and extend it upwards. The arm movement carries your fist up to head height, well away from your body. As you can see in the illustration, the arm remains relaxed with a slight curve.

Your left arm also rises up naturally, reaching head height as well, but not extended outwards. Your shoulders remain relaxed.

Once you become familiar with this upward explosive motion, change the position of your feet: turn one foot 45 degrees outwards and step forwards with the other. Train with your feet and arms in the reverse order so that you can make the swing comfortably to both diagonals.

Begin gradually to fully understand the loose, upward bounce of your arms. The action should be light and unrestrained. Start slowly. Build up to 30 times. When you can do the movement repeatedly without being held back by tension, practice as much as you wish.

9

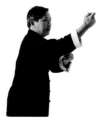

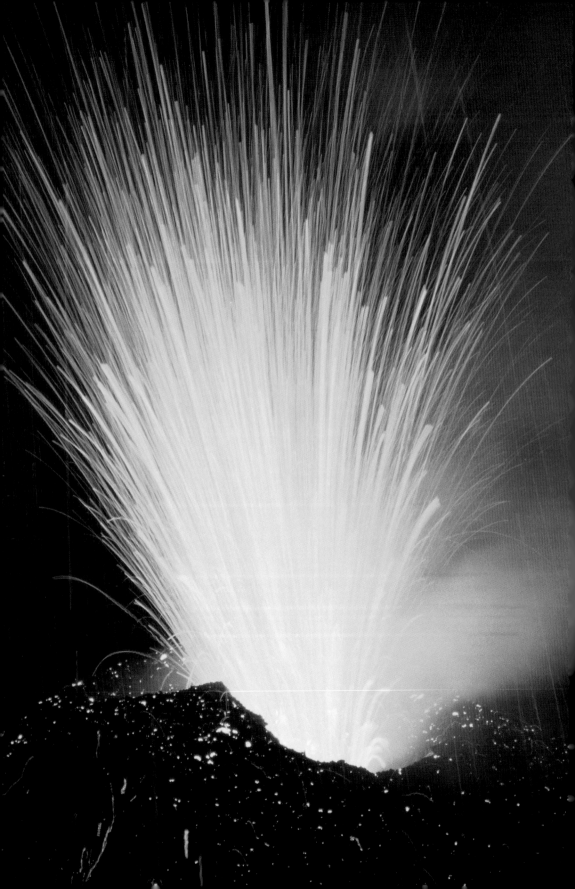

Fire Power

Fire is the energy we most commonly associate with explosive power. Its intensity is matched by its speed. Its power radiates outwards with the brilliance and velocity of light.

In the words of Grand Master Wang Xiang Zhai: "Fire means having the strength of gunpowder, fists like bullets, the strength to bury your opponent at the first touch."

This movement begins in the depths of your being and travels upwards. It begins in the Sea of Chi, your lower Tan Tien. The motion starts with the movement of your hips and the power is finally expressed through the upper thrust of your hands.

You need to be completely free from any obstructing tension that could block the release of energy. At first, your power will be blocked by tension at many points – as surely as hardened fire doors retard the spread of flames. This is why it is essential for all who aspire to master this art to train constantly in inner relaxation and the release of tension.

When you make progress, the twist of your body and the upward burst of your hands becomes like an explosion. Like a volcano erupting through the earth, unrestrained power surges through your fists. They become like leather whips snapping with full strength.

The Fire Power of the human being is indispensable. Without it we become lifeless. Training to release this energy affects us on many levels. It burns off physical, mental and emotional obstructions, from muscle tension to sluggishness and depression. It develops our personal warmth, humor and creativity. It is the essence of intuitive power, vision and imagination.

10

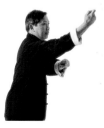

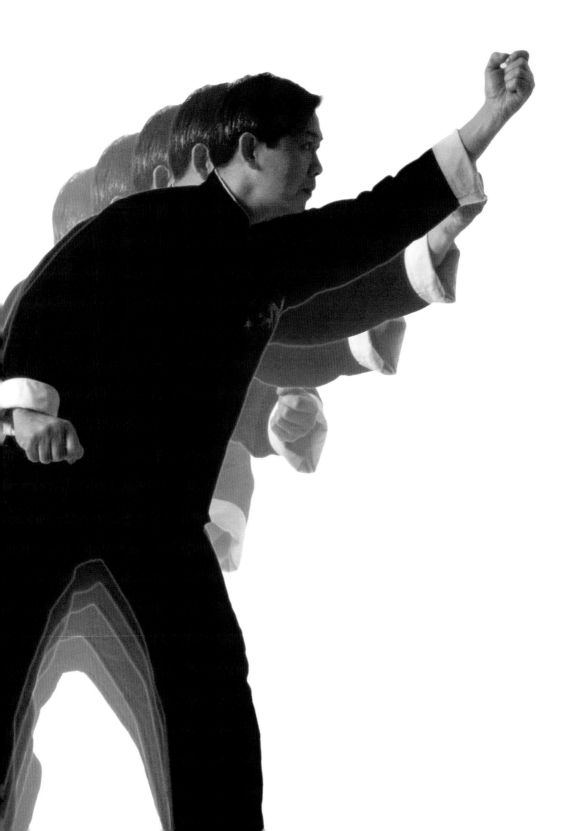

Earth 土

Begin your training in Wu Chi. Feel the weight of your body firmly on the soles of your feet and let any tension in your shoulders, neck, chest and hips drain away. Then slowly raise your arms into the position, Holding the Belly (page 13), with your arms gently curved as if resting on a very full abdomen, like the belly of The Laughing Buddha.

Fold your hands into loose fists, making an arrowhead on each one, as you can clearly see on the facing page.

Move your arms apart in opposite directions, one to the left, one to the right. One moves upwards in the direction of the upper diagonal. The other moves downwards in the direction of the lower diagonal. Then bring them back in towards you and strike outwards to the opposite diagonals.

Imagine you are striking steel bars on either side of you with full force, using the edges of your forearms and fists. Practice directing your energy to both sides, striking first the upper left diagonal with your left forearm and the lower right diagonal with your right forearm and then the opposite diagonals with the opposite arms.

Once you become familiar with the diagonal splitting motion, change the position of your feet: turn one foot 45 degrees outwards and step forwards with the other. Look straight ahead and continue to strike the diagonals with your forearms.

Begin gradually and pay attention to the correct movement of your arms. The action should be smooth and relaxed. Start slowly. Build up to 30 times. When you can comfortably do the movement without tensing your chest or shoulders, practice as much as you wish.

11

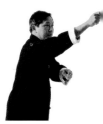

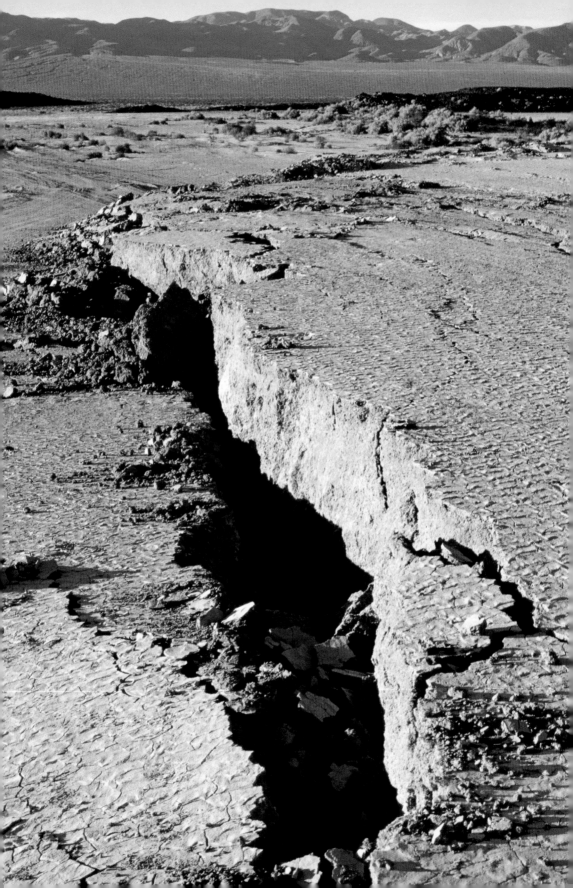

Earth Power

In the system of the Five Energies, Earth is considered the pivot, the central fulcrum around which the others move in a constant interchange. Like planet earth itself, this energy has tremendous depth and stability. It has all the qualities of a sphere, perfectly round, perfectly balanced. It is like a mountain in its power – able to absorb other forces and sustain all forms of life.

In the words of Grand Master Wang Xiang Zhai: "Earth exerts strength that is heavy, deep, solid and perfectly round. The Chi is being strong, having the power of heaven and earth in harmony with each other."

When you first learn this movement, you feel your arms are expanding to the sides, making a sharp diagonal line across the front of your body. This feeling of straightness comes from your inner tension. As you develop the true relaxed power of the movement, you perceive the curving quality of the motion.

The circular, sweeping power of this motion is like a heavy scythe swinging with full force through a field of wheat. Like a storm, it slices across the grain in wide, deadly arcs. As you learn to express this power more fully, your arms become like the coiling tails of huge reptiles. Like a crocodile sweeping and swaying from side to side, your power uproots and crushes whatever is hit.

Earth Power is greater than the earth itself. It is the power that cracks the earth apart.

That power is within you. It is expansive, gives you great stability, is the source of acceptance and flexibility under even the most difficult of circumstances. It gives you balance and depth. But when the time comes for you to express your deepest feelings, to open your heart or to break through old habits of mind, you will find within you the power of an earthquake.

12

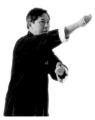

Your Natural Strength: Sports

Da Cheng Chuan strengthens your body and sharpens your mind. It increases your stamina and endurance. It takes you beyond your normal limits and helps protect you against injury.

Champions need to set their sights far beyond what they might normally achieve, and must develop unusually high levels of stamina. The advanced practices in this book take you beyond the barrier of pain, awaken muscles and nerves previously dormant and help you remain relaxed while exerting yourself to the maximum.

The art of Da Cheng Chuan, from its foundations in Wu Chi through to its pinnacle in combat, is really a training in personal bravery. Freedom from fear is essential. Explaining this to his students, Professor Yu is fond of quoting the great sage Lao Tse: "Those who have tempered themselves are not afraid of encountering tigers."

As Zhan Zhuang works on your entire energy field it helps to break the vicious cycle of nervousness and physical tension. The benefits of your training will start to show themselves in those moments that require concentration and relaxation at the same time, such as hitting a golf ball, serving a match point in tennis or scoring a goal in soccer.

Professor Yu emphasizes the physical benefits, too: "It is important to know how to relieve stress when your muscles are overstimulated, otherwise they will remain tense and you will tire rapidly. If you have mastered the technique of relaxation, you use much less energy and do not suffer from rapid fatigue." The training in muscular contraction and relaxation (pages 88–89) automatically develops this skill.

Having mastered the foundations and done your warm-up exercises, you should pay particular emphasis to going as low as possible in the postures. Take care not to let your knees bend forwards over your toes. If you feel pain or trembling in the legs, relieve it by going still lower! While holding the deep positions, scan your upper body for tension and relax whatever muscles have tightened. You will need to repeat the scanning and relaxation constantly, until you feel that all the work is being done in your legs, leaving your torso and head to rest free and easy in the position.

"Red triangle" training (pages 84–85) also yields excellent sports results. In addition to standing with your weight balanced only on the triangles, contract your calf muscles so that they are as firm as rocks. Grip the floor firmly with your toes. Grip and tense for ten seconds, then relax – repeating this sequence up to 30 times, with your upper body completely relaxed.

You can also continue your training when out walking: feel as if you are going up

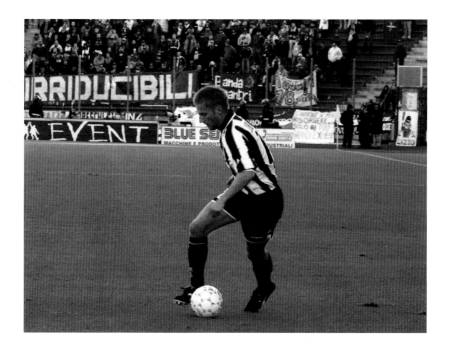

an incline, secretly using your "red triangles" to increase your power.

The lower body power developed by Da Cheng Chuan can make a difference in almost every sport. For example, in equestrian sports it gives riders exactly the control they need in the stirrups, with balance and freedom in the upper body. In sports that demand precise synchro-nization of mind and body, it stabilizes the entire body structure while training the central nervous system. In body contact sports, the powerful energy field developed by Da Cheng Chuan acts as a protective shield against injury, while sharpening and extending the competitor's range of awareness.

As its benefits become better known, Da Cheng Chuan training is finding its way into the sports world outside China. For example, Martin Jørgensen (pictured above playing for the Italian soccer team, Udinese) is a Danish athlete who has been studying Da Cheng Chuan for years. He uses it regularly in his work-out routines and stands like a tree in the breaks during games!

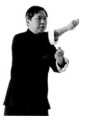

13

THE GREAT ACCOMPLISHMENT LINEAGE IV

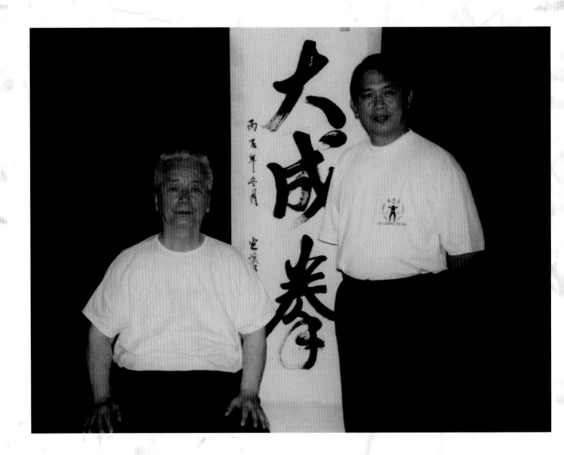

One of the earliest students of Grand Master Wang Xiang Zhai was a young man who had studied orthodox Western medicine and then specialized in dentistry. His name was Yu Yong Nian.

Yu Yong Nian was born near Beijing in February 1920. After completing his initial schooling he was sent for specialist medical education in Japan. At 21, he returned to China and began work at the Beijing Railway General Hospital.

Three years later, exhausted from the long, constant hours of dental practice, he began training under Grand Master Wang Xiang Zhai. After nine years' study and practice, Yu Yong Nian began to introduce aspects of Zhan Zhuang as treatment for internal diseases at his hospital. His initial successes led to a major medical conference in 1956 at the Beijing Shoudong San Hospital to introduce the Zhan Zhuang system to hospitals throughout China.

"When I was training in the park under Master Wang Xiang Zhai," Professor Yu later recalled, "he would tell me to 'pull the tree' towards me and then push it back. This was from a distance and I couldn't imagine how I could possibly do that! I tried every day. Only after long practice did I begin to feel the connection with the tree. Then I began to understand his words."

After the Cultural Revolution, Professor Yu published the first of four books on the Zhan Zhuang system. The first edition of *Zhan Zhuang for Health* (Educational Publishers, Beijing) was published in February 1982 with a print run of 20,000 copies. By April, a second edition of 120,000 copies was issued. By 1987, a further 294,500 copies had been printed.

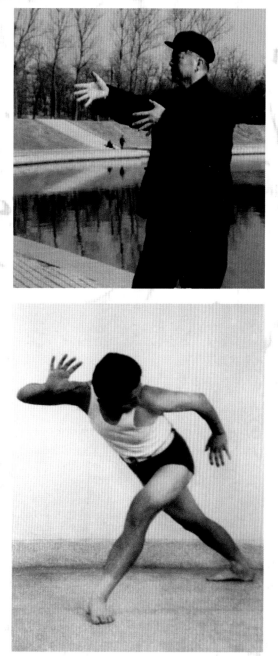

A limited edition of his second book on the application of Zhan Zhuang for health was published in Beijing in 1989 and in the same year a further book on the system was issued by Cosmos Books in Hong Kong.

Professor Yu, now the world's leading authority on Zhan Zhuang Chi Kung, is a member of China's National Chi Kung Research Council. He is also consultant to the American-Chinese Chi Kung Research Group and consultant to the Da Cheng Chuan Zhan Zhuang Chi Kung Research Groups (Europe).

混沌恍惚乾坤內歛

毛髮舒張精炁鼓盪

持環得樞風雷雨電

山吼海嘯芽盾渾圓

錦全

THE
CIRCLE OF
HARMONY

Calligraphy by Master Lam Kam Chuen,
described in the introduction to Part Five.

The beginning of all things is invisible:
At first, there is only a pulse.
Every hair is fully alert –
Wind, thunder, rain, lightning.
The mountain roars,
The ocean boils.
Spear and shield,
Harmonized in one circle –
This is the great accomplishment.

The original calligraphy of these lines is reproduced on the opening page of Part Five (page 132). I composed these lines to express my own understanding of the profound wisdom of Da Cheng Chuan.

The wellsprings of this art lie in the Taoist tradition. "Knowing the ancient beginning is the essence of the Way," wrote the great sage Lao Tse. Our ancestors drew a perfect circle to symbolize the beginning of everything – an unfertilized egg, unseen yet filled with the potential of life. At the instant of conception there is a single pulse of energy, like the movement of a microscopic sperm. In exactly the same way, motion is born of stillness through The Great Accomplishment.

In the fully energized state, "every hair is fully alert." The state of relaxed arousal is what is meant by the Chinese term "sung." This is not the drowsy torpor before sleep. It is the release of tension that saps our strength – so that we become alert, clear-headed and full of vigor. Your head is uplifted and your eyes open, while letting go of the physical tension in your muscles and organs.

The full power of your energy moves like the forces of nature: "wind, thunder, rain and lightning." As your Chi circulates inside you and radiates outwards, it hammers through any obstacles. You feel like a mountain shuddering. To an opponent, your force is like a roar.

The power of Chi generates heat throughout your being: just as in the ancient Chinese ideogram, the fire boils the water. Deep within the ocean of your being, your Chi begins to stir and you feel its vibrations in your bloodstream.

The spear and shield, as in much Chinese poetry, have multiple meanings. Together, they refer to the martial application of this art. They describe the Zhan Zhuang position – one hand curved in front as a shield, the other pointed forwards as a spear – shown on page 50 . They are the symbols of attack and defense, the twin polarities of the martial arts.

"Harmonized in one circle" expresses the complete view of Da Cheng Chuan, which is also described by the Chinese term "wunyuanzhuang" – the perfect circle. Your being, like a great sphere, is totally pervaded with energy, the ultimate accomplishment of this art. At its pinnacle, Da Cheng Chuan fuses all the elements – physical, mental and spiritual, as well as its health and martial applications – into a perfect whole.

Your introduction to this system is completed in Part Five as you learn a series of foot movements that can be combined with the postures and arm movements for in-depth training.

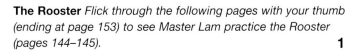

The Rooster *Flick through the following pages with your thumb (ending at page 153) to see Master Lam practice the Rooster (pages 144–145).* **1**

Power Testing

One of the distinctive practices of Da Cheng Chuan is known as Shih Li, traditionally translated as "power testing." These slow, careful movements take place on one spot. They involve the movement of the whole body and are an indispensable part of the martial arts training. They can also be practiced to develop skillful synchronization of mind and body.

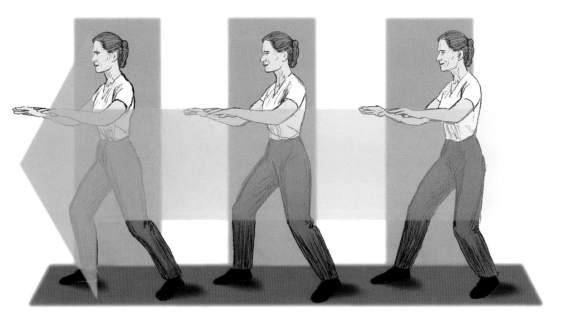

Stand with your feet shoulder width apart. Turn your left foot 45 degrees outwards. Move your right foot forwards, pointing straight ahead. Lower yourself as far as possible over your rear leg. Slowly shift forwards until all your weight is over your front foot, with your front calf perpendicular to the ground. Take care that your knee never extends forwards beyond your toes.

Breathe out when you move forwards. Breathe in when you move backwards.

As your body moves forwards, your forearms are extended
in front of you, your palms facing down, your fingers pointing
forwards. You imagine you are pushing a heavy weight forwards
with your fingertips. When your body moves backwards, your
hands turn so that your palms face each other. You imagine you
are pulling a heavy weight towards you. The angles of your
elbows remain constant.

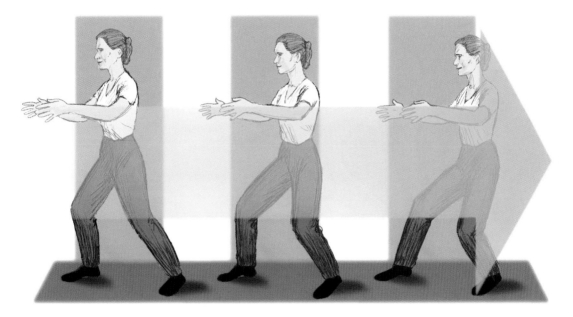

Once your weight is fully forwards, you start to shift slowly
backwards. As you move, your body remains level. The even
movement forwards and backwards is carefully controlled
through your knees, with all weight concentrated in your lower
body. Your upper body and arms remain relaxed throughout.

2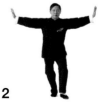

Tortoise in the Sea

This is a more advanced Shih Li practice. It takes its name from the motion of a tortoise swimming up to the surface of the sea and using its front flippers to keep its head above the water. As you develop your understanding of the motion, you have the feeling of a large bellows opening and closing with great power. To begin, move into the On Guard position (pages 36–37). Keep the heel of your front foot slightly raised off the ground throughout this exercise.

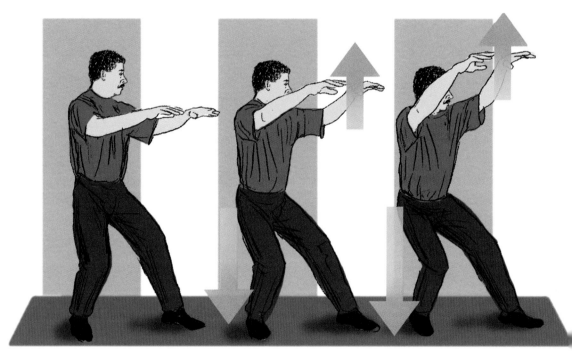

Slowly sink your weight down over your rear leg. Take care not to stick your bottom out backwards. As your weight sinks down, both your arms gently rise up until they are level with the top of your head. Your upper body and arms remain relaxed and there is a gentle curve in your elbows. As you sink down, breathe in.

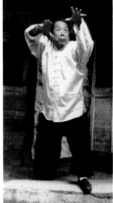

Master Wang Xuan Jie, an accomplished Da Cheng Chuan practitioner, demonstrates the Tortoise in the Sea. He keeps his weight on his rear leg, practicing with his front foot on a step. You can clearly see the open spread of his fingers – one of the signatures of this art.

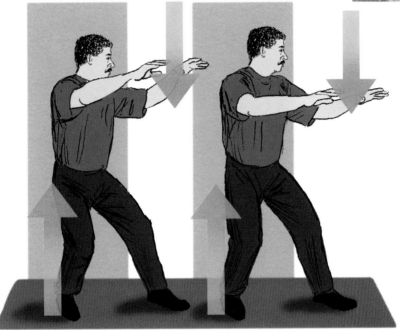

When you have gone as low as you can over the rear leg, start to rise slowly up. This motion feels as if it is driven entirely from a hydraulic pump in your rear leg. As you rise up, your arms move downwards at the same slow speed to their original position. Breathe out with this phase of the motion.

3

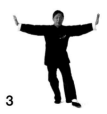

Ice Step

Once you have learned the Zhan Zhuang standing positions in
Parts One and Two of this book, you can begin to practice the
specialized steps used in Da Cheng Chuan. The first movement
is called the Ice Step because it evokes the feeling of someone
slowly and carefully making their way across the surface of a
frozen pond. It improves your kinesthetic control and develops
your balance.

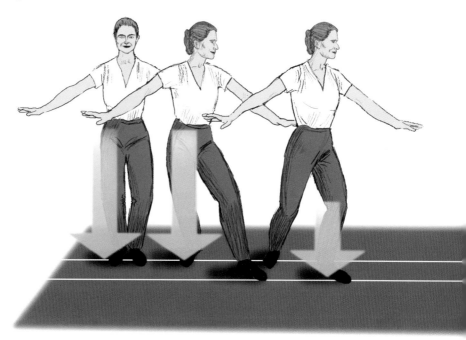

Stand with your feet together, your knees slightly bent. Shift all
your weight onto one foot. Imagine the floor is made of ice.
Keeping your weight entirely on one side, move your other foot
forwards in an arc over the surface of the ice. The sole of your
foot is about a centimeter (half an inch) above the ice.

Then lower the extended foot on to the ice and slowly shift all
your weight forwards on to that foot. Breathe out as your weight
moves forwards.

You can hold your arms in each of the Zhan Zhuang positions while practicing the Ice Step. To begin, your balance will be best if you hold your arms in the posture, Extending to the Sides (page 14). Your arms are calmly extended to either side. Your hands are relaxed and open. Your upper body is upright without tension.

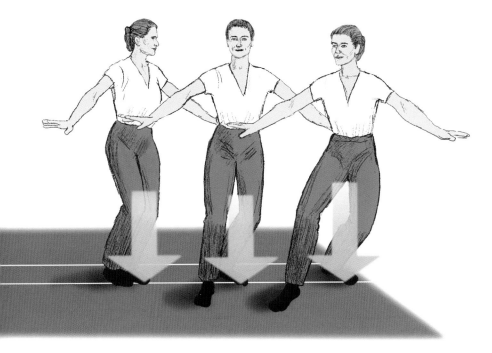

Slowly bring your rear foot up into position beside your front foot. As you move your foot, the sole stays parallel to the ice, a centimeter (half an inch) above the surface. Breathe in as you bring your foot into position beside the stationary one. You are now ready to move it forwards in an arc over the ice. Continue alternating your feet in the Ice Step as you move across the ice.

4

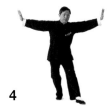

Xing Yi

This step comes from the martial art Xing Yi, which Grand
Master Wang Xiang Zhai learned from his first teacher, Master
Guo Yun Sin. To begin, stand in the Zhan Zhuang position,
Holding the Ball (page 13). Shift all your weight on to one foot.
Swivel your other foot on the heel 90 degrees to point sideways.
It is now pointing in the forward direction in which you will move.

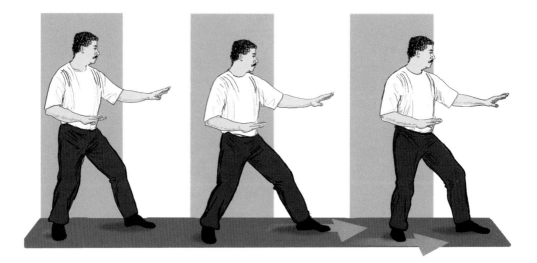

Your feet are at right angles to each other. All your weight is
on your rear foot. Keeping your rear foot firmly in position, step
slightly forwards with your front foot, without shifting any weight
on to it. Then bring the rear foot slightly towards the front foot
and plant it firmly on the ground, still bearing all your weight.
The distance between your two feet is now the same as when
you began.

Breathe in as you place your front foot forwards. Breathe out as
you move your rear foot forwards.

When you practice this step, you can hold your arms in any of the Zhan Zhuang positions you have learned. To begin, the most common arm position with this step is the On Guard position (pages 36–37). When your right foot is moving forwards, your right hand points in the same direction. Likewise, when your left foot moves forwards, your left hand points in the same direction.

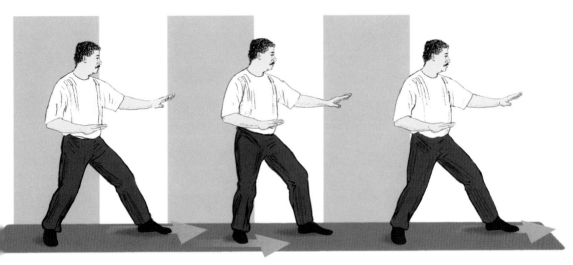

Apart from the tiny forward movements of the front foot, all the work is done by the muscles of the rear leg. As you practice, try not to hop up and down too much on your rear leg. The movement should be silent. Stay low and level, slowly inching forwards using the power of your rear leg.

5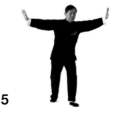

The Rooster

Many movements in the Chinese martial arts are drawn from close observation of nature. This step resembles the motion of a rooster as it places its feet deliberately and powerfully on the ground. It is an energizing exercise in itself and is used in the martial application of Da Cheng Chuan to conquer the ground from an opponent.

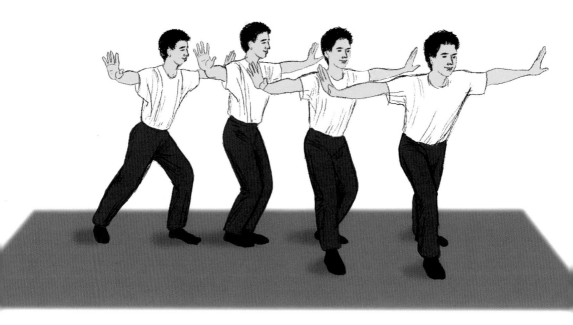

Start with your feet together, knees bent, weight on one foot. Extend your arms fully to the sides, palms facing away from you, fingers up. Move your free foot forwards in an arc out to the diagonal. Keep the sole of your foot parallel to the ground and a centimeter (half an inch) off it.

Place your foot flat on the ground and slowly lean over it until your weight is fully forwards. Breathe out as you do this.

As you practice The Rooster, the orientation of your upper body changes with each step. You move from diagonal to diagonal. First you face towards one diagonal and lean forwards over your front foot in that direction. Then, when you are ready to begin the next step, your hips turn so that you are facing the other diagonal before you step forwards.

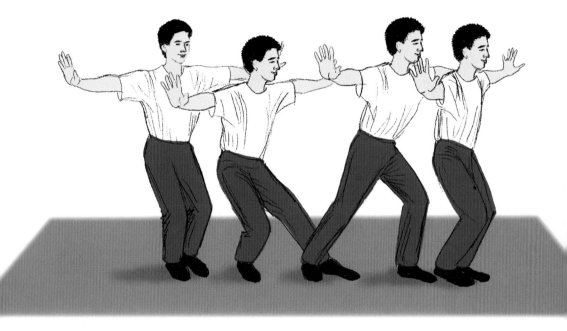

Bring your rear foot slowly up to your front foot. Move it so that the sole remains parallel to the ground and a centimeter (half an inch) off it. Your body straightens up as you rest the ball of the foot on the ground beside your other foot. Breathe in as you straighten up. Then continue with the next step of The Rooster.

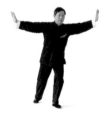

6

The Bear

This movement is for Da Cheng Chuan practitioners who have reached a reasonably high level of accomplishment. Outwardly, the movement appears to be very slight. However, it requires a great deal of bodily control and considerable inner strength. Its power in combat is immense.

When this movement is practiced properly, the person moves forward like a bear rearing up on its hind legs ready to brush away anything in its path.

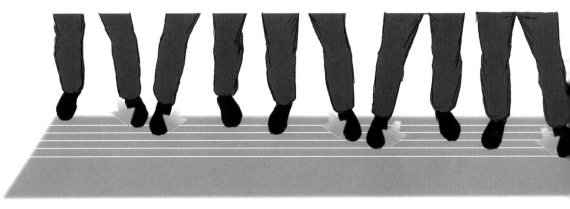

Stand with your feet facing forwards and shoulder width apart. Spread your weight evenly over both feet. Take a small step forwards with one foot, no more than 5 cm (2 in). Lift and place your foot so that the sole is always parallel to the ground. It feels as if the entire movement comes from the back of your leg. Take care not to shift your weight from one side to the other as you move.

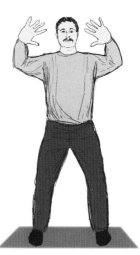

This movement is normally accompanied by the arm position featured in Opening Outwards (page 14).

Your arms are fully relaxed, with your hands opening outwards in front of your head. Your fingers are spread apart like the claws of a bear.

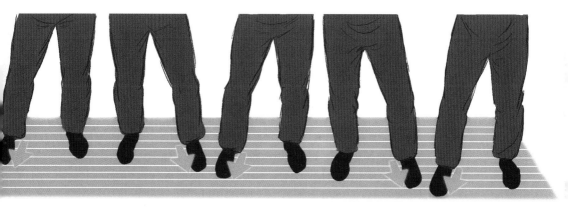

As you move forwards, making small steps, the center line of your body remains stable. This is unlike normal walking: there is no lateral shifting of the body weight. Once you start to understand the inner mechanics of this movement, try to synchronize your breathing with it. Breathe out with each forward step.

7

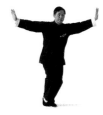

The Five Signs of Practice

*When you look at a person who is a Zhan Zhuang
practitioner, you can assess their development
according to the Five Signs.
First is the person's Form. This refers to their posture: are they
holding themselves in the correct positions?
Second is the person's Mind. Are they present and paying
attention to their practice or are they literally "absent-minded"?
Third is the person's Power.
Is there dynamism in the way they stand?
Fourth is Energy. Is there a sense that energy is emanating
from them, like an aura?
Fifth is the Spirit. Does the person manifest the quality of
being an antenna raised between the two powers of Earth
and Heaven. All these should come together.*

Professor Yu Yong Nian

Your training is a gradual process of development. It never ends.
There is no limit to it. In conventional physical exercise, there is
always some limit imposed by the human body. But in Zhan
Zhuang, we continue to train our body, mind and spirit as a unity.

Daily practice is the key. The framework charts on these pages
will help you. Remember that the foundation at all levels is the
standing practice of Zhan Zhuang. Add movement training only
after your daily standing practice.

It is always best to train under the guidance of a qualified
instructor. If this is not possible, follow the instructions in this
book with great care. It is extremely important not to rush your
training or to push yourself beyond your own natural endurance.
Always remember the words of Grand Master Wang Xiang Zhai:

*Keep on practicing like this with perseverance
The skill will come to you of itself.*

First Level If you are beginning this practice for the first time, or have only been practicing Zhan Zhuang for a year or less, you should develop a daily routine. Your daily framework is shown in the chart below. Start with the three warm-up exercises, stand in Wu Chi, then practice one of the foundation postures. Build up to 15 minutes without moving and close by Sealing your Energy.

FRAMEWORK	EXERCISE	PAGE	NUMBERS/DURATION
WARM-UPS	Relaxing the Shoulders	11	*30 circles*
	Rotating the Hips	11	*30 each way*
	Strengthening the Knees	11	*30 each way*
	Wu Chi	26–27	*5 mins up to 15 mins*
FOUNDATION POSTURES	Holding the Belly	13	*5 mins up to 15 mins*
	Holding the Ball	13	*5 mins up to 15 mins*
	Extending to the Sides	14	*5 mins up to 15 mins*
	Opening Outwards	14	*5 mins up to 15 mins*
CLOSING PRACTICE	Wu Chi	26–27	*2 to 5 mins*
	Sealing your Energy	15	*2 to 5 mins*

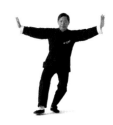

8

Second Level   If you have reached the point in your practice where you can stand for 15 minutes in each of the foundation postures, experiment with the next level shown in the chart below. The framework for this level is the warm-ups with new additions, standing in Wu Chi and the postures shown in Part One (gradually going lower in each posture). You always close by standing in Wu Chi and Sealing your Energy.

FRAMEWORK	EXERCISE	PAGE	NUMBER/DURATION
WARM-UPS	Relaxing the Shoulders	11	*30 circles*
	Rotating the Hips	11	*30 each way*
	Strengthening the Knees	11	*30 each way*
NEW WARM-UPS	Opening the Inner Gate	20–21	*10 up to 30*
	Arm Circles	22–23	*10 up to 30*
	Knees Up	24–25	*10 up to 30*
	Wu Chi	26–27	*5 mins up to 20 mins*
PART ONE POSTURES	The Great Circle	28–29	*go deeper; stay longer*
	Double Spirals	30–31	*go deeper; stay longer*
	On Guard	36–37	*go deeper; stay longer*
	Dragon Mouth	38–39	*go deeper; stay longer*
CLOSING PRACTICE	Wu Chi	26-27	*2 to 5 mins*
	Sealing your Energy	15	*2 to 5 mins*

Third Level   If you have reached the point in your daily practice where you are doing the maximum numbers for all the warm-ups in Level Two, and are reasonably stable holding the postures at least 10 cm (5 in) lower than your normal standing height, you can experiment with a more advanced routine shown in the chart below.

FRAMEWORK	EXERCISE	PAGE	NUMBER/DURATION
WARM-UPS	Opening the Inner Gate	20–21	*30 up to 60*
	Arm Circles	22–23	*30 up to 60*
	Knees Up	24–25	*30 up to 60*
	Full Swing	106–107	*30 up to 60*
	Wu Chi	26–27	*5 mins up to 20 mins*
VARIOUS POSTURES	The Great Circle	28–29	*go deeper; stay longer*
	Double Spirals	30–31	*go deeper; stay longer*
	The Archer	48–49	*go deeper; stay longer*
	The Dragon	56–59	*go deeper; stay longer*
	Holding the Tiger	60–63	*go deeper; stay longer*
MOVEMENTS	A power movement from Part Four		*5 mins or longer*
	One of the steps in Part Five		*5 mins or longer*
CLOSING PRACTICE	Wu Chi	26–27	*2 to 5 mins*
	Sealing your Energy	15	*2 to 5 mins*

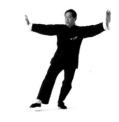

9

Your Natural Strength: Creativity

Your creativity is a natural expression of your energy. When you cultivate your inner power, you are opening up your ability to work with the tremendous energy that surrounds you. This is the secret of the living arts, from parenting and cooking to singing, dancing and all the other performing arts.

Your daily practice gradually enables your Chi to flow smoothly through your system. It opens your mind and heart and develops your sensitivity. You begin to be more intuitive and perceptive. You experience higher levels of energy, and are less nervous in the midst of swirling movement and emotion.

In classical Chinese culture, the mastery of integrating stillness and motion is seen in the work of the great calligraphers. It's no surprise that Master Li Jian Yu, one of the oldest and most respected calligraphers still working today, studied directly under Grand Master Wang Xiang Zhai in Beijing. He is seen at his art on the facing page. Master Li's calligraphy of Da Cheng Chuan opens this book.

"Grand Master Wang was very calm and elegant," recalls Master Li. "When you saw him like that, it was difficult to imagine that he was a practitioner of Chinese boxing. He was not only concerned with daily physical training. He wanted us to have a correct vision of the world, seeing things from different angles. He often talked to me about philosophy."

Musicians and performing artists who are my students have told me how Zhan Zhuang helped their art. One of my European students is a classical singer, Monika Riedler (seen on stage in an opera below). She says: "Zhan Zhuang has extended my capacity. The change is fundamental: you can hear the difference. I am stronger, breathe deeper and project my voice further. Zhan Zhuang has changed my awareness of my inner space. I couldn't have learned this just from taking singing lessons."

"Zhan Zhuang is the best possible training for anyone working with a musical instrument," declares pianist and teacher, Robin Rubenstein. "My

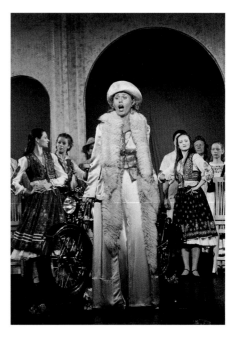

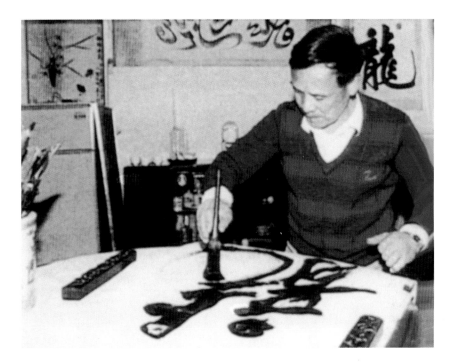

experience of the music is far deeper. Instead of using up my energy, I feel I am releasing it – the instrument becomes my voice. Performing takes less out of me physically and I no longer have the same nervous tension. I feel the power flowing from my body through my arms into the keyboard." Composer and violinist Wilfred Gibson agrees: "It's like riding a horse. You feel you are working with that power. If I spend nine hours in a recording studio, I do half an hour of Zhan Zhuang in the lunch break. Then even when everyone else is flagging, I find I have a reserve of energy I can draw on."

Grand Master Wang Xiang Zhai took a great interest in all manner of arts. The imagery in his poetry reflects his own creativity. Whatever you do, remember that the possibilities of your energy are limitless. In the words of Grand Master Wang:

*With your heroic spirit you can shake
both heaven and earth
With a broad mind, you have all the
universe in your mind.*

10

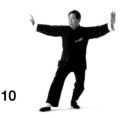

THE GREAT ACCOMPLISHMENT LINEAGE V

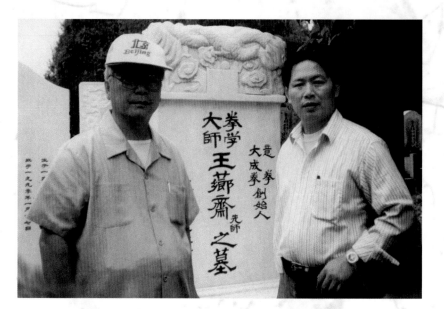

Professor Yu Yong Nian maintained the spread of this art through his teaching and best-selling books. In the late 1960s, a newspaper article that appeared about him in China made its way into the hands of a young martial artist in Hong Kong, Lam Kam Chuen.

He had already been introduced to Da Cheng Chuan through a Buddhist master, but now he had found a way to contact a teacher who had studied directly under Grand Master Wang Xiang Zhai. For years it was only possible for him to correspond with Professor Yu until, towards the end of China's Cultural Revolution, he was finally able to travel to Beijing and be accepted as a student.

After a decade of advanced study, Master Lam was accorded the honor of being acknowledged as a lineage-holder of the Da Cheng Chuan tradition by Madame Wang Yuk Fong (page 74), the daughter and spiritual heir of Grand Master Wang Xiang Zhai.

Master Lam Kam Chuen has continued to work closely with Professor Yu. It is a professional collaboration that spans the Western medical system – in which Professor Yu trained as dental surgeon – and Traditional Chinese Medicine, which Master Lam practices. Their extensive yet distinct medical experience is unified by their common practice of Chi Kung.

After coming to the West, Master Lam gave the first European demonstration of Da Cheng Chuan before a capacity audience in London in 1987. He then received permission from Professor Yu

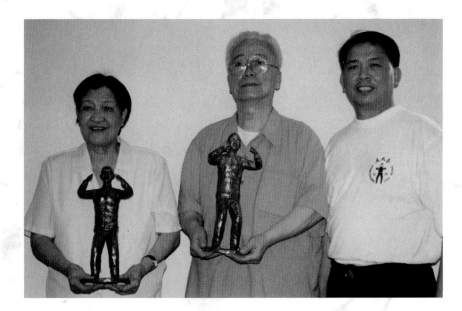

to commence training students in the art. This was followed by his ground-breaking work *The Way of Energy*, which introduces Zhan Zhuang to the West and to which Professor Yu wrote a foreword. The book has now been translated into more than a dozen languages, selling tens of thousands of copies worldwide.

In 1994, he was invited by UK television network Channel 4 to present a ten-part series *Stand Still Be Fit*, filmed on location in China and Hong Kong. Public response was unprecedented, with thousands ordering copies of the instruction booklet that accompanied the series.

Master Lam continues to teach and travel widely in Europe and North America. He regularly arranges visits,

teaching programs and seminars that enable Western students to train under Chinese masters and exchange experience with practitioners in China.

The Western students who first trained to become instructors are holders of the limited-edition statue of Grand Master Wang Xiang Zhai, held by Professor Yu and Madame Wang in the photo above.

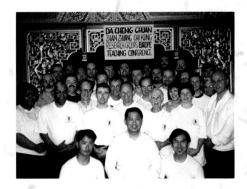

About the Author

Master Lam Kam Chuen has devoted his life to the classical arts of Chinese culture. He has brought these to the West, introducing Chinese health care to millions through his books, videos and TV appearances.

A living example of Chinese holistic culture, Master Lam is accomplished in the "Five Arts" studied by the advisers to the imperial court. The Five Arts – San, Yi, Ming, Bok and Shang – comprise the Taoist and Buddhist arts, systems for internal medicine and health exercise, Feng Shui, astrology and the interpretation of the *I Ching*.

Master Lam's life-long study has brought together many strands of China's martial arts heritage. These influences are reflected in his own style of Da Cheng Chuan, presented in this book, and the methods he uses to teach Western students.

A summary of the martial arts studied by Master Lam, along with the lines of their teaching lineages, is shown opposite.

Master Lam began his formal martial arts instruction at the age of 11, training in Xing Yi under 80-year-old Master Fung in Hong Kong. He then studied the techniques that were handed down by the Shaolin Temple lineages under Master Leung Tse Cheung and Master Kim Sheung Mo. Both were disciples of Grand Master Ku Yue Chang, at that time the "King of Iron Palm" in China.

As a member of the Hong Kong Chinese Martial Arts Association, he went on to victory in tournaments in Hong Kong and Taiwan and in the Southeast Asia Open Tournament in Malaysia.

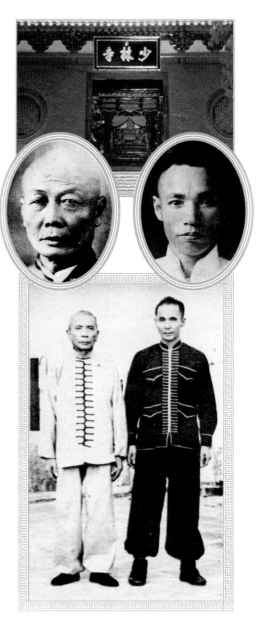

Above top: Shaolin Temple gateway. Middle left and right: Choy Lee Fut Master Tan San, Master Ku Yue Chang. Bottom left and right: Master Kim Sheung Mo, Master Leung Tse Cheung.

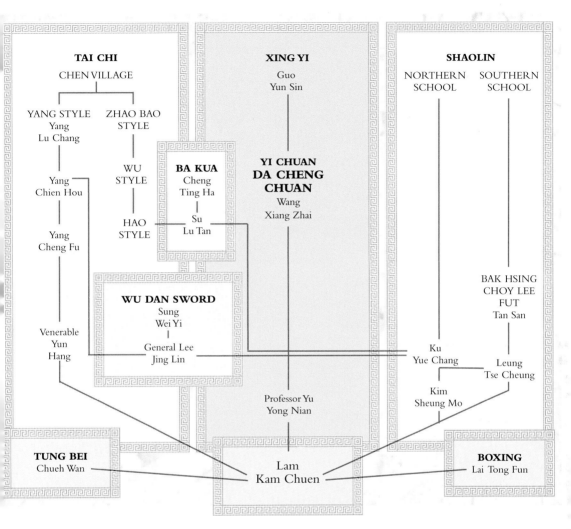

TAI CHI
CHEN VILLAGE

YANG STYLE
Yang
Lu Chang

ZHAO BAO
STYLE

WU
STYLE

HAO
STYLE

Yang
Chien Hou

Yang
Cheng Fu

Venerable
Yun
Hang

BA KUA
Cheng
Ting Ha

Su
Lu Tan

XING YI
Guo
Yun Sin

**YI CHUAN
DA CHENG
CHUAN**
Wang
Xiang Zhai

SHAOLIN
NORTHERN   SOUTHERN
SCHOOL   SCHOOL

BAK HSING
CHOY LEE
FUT
Tan San

WU DAN SWORD
Sung
Wei Yi

General Lee
Jing Lin

Ku
Yue Chang

Leung
Tse Cheung

Kim
Sheung Mo

Professor Yu
Yong Nian

TUNG BEI
Chueh Wan

Lam
Kam Chuen

BOXING
Lai Tong Fun

As part of his deep training in the martial arts, Master Lam learned the Old Sun Style of Tai Chi from Master Leung Tse Cheung, as well as Choy Lee Fut, Iron Palm and the use of the sword and spear. Fusing this early training with later studies in the internal art of Chi Kung, Master Lam Kam Chuen has since developed his own internationally recognized Tai Chi tradition: Lam Style Tai Chi Chuan.

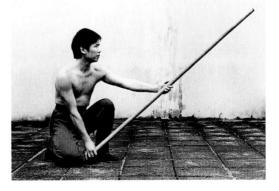

The young Lam Kam Chuen practicing Shaolin Pole.

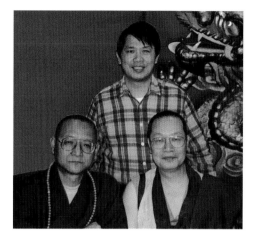

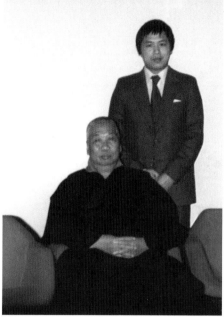

Above: Master Lam with the Venerable Yeung Quen and Master Lau Sau Hong. Right: seated in foreground, the Venerable Master Yun Hang.

Master Lam is a highly accomplished practitioner of Traditional Chinese Medicine, having qualified at an early age as a herbalist and bone-setter, and establishing his own health clinic and martial arts school in Hong Kong.

The turning point in Master Lam's career was his introduction to a Yi Chuan master, who had trained in the tradition of Grand Master Wang Xiang Zhai. "By testing myself against this master, I found that his system was far more powerful than anything I had learned already," Master Lam recalls. "After this I changed everything, using the forms I already knew but with a new power that gave my martial arts new life."

Master Lam's training also immersed him in the Taoist and Buddhist traditions. It was a Buddhist Master, Lau Sau Hong, who introduced him to the art of Wang Xiang Zhai and to a senior Chinese Vajrayana Buddhist teacher, Master Yun Hang, under whom

Master Lam undertook advanced Buddhist studies. While Master Yun Hang was alive, he transmitted to Master Lam a series of teachings which he had personally received from Tai Chi Master Yang Cheng Fu.

In 1975, Master Lam, newly married to another martial artist, Lam Kai Sin, came to the United Kingdom. He accepted an invitation to teach Taoist Arts at the Mary Ward Centre in London, and has remained in the United Kingdom ever since. Thanks to his efforts, Tai Chi was accepted as a legitimate subject for the adult education curriculum of the Inner London Education Authority, clearing the way for the teaching of this art to thousands of Londoners and others throughout the United Kingdom. He continues to teach, and is nurturing the art of Da Cheng Chuan with a small number of experienced students and trainee teachers across Europe.

FURTHER TRAINING

Da Cheng Chuan has seven stages. This book introduces you to the first three. First is Zhan Zhuang, or Standing Like a Tree. Next is Shih Li, or Power Testing, followed by Tsou Pu, or Step Training. Practitioners then cultivate the explosive power of Fa Li or Fa Jing. The fifth stage is Tui Shou, or Circling Hands, which involves training with a partner and is often called Pushing Hands. Next, the student undertakes the freestyle combat of Shih Zhan. At the highest level the practitioner learns Jian Wu, the display of spontaneous power.

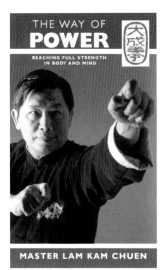

The Way of Power video complements the instructions in this book. For further information about the video, Zhan Zhuang classes and workshops, please visit our website: www.lamassociation.org. You can contact The Lam Association at 1 Hercules Road, London SE1 7DP. Tel/Fax: (+44) 020 7261 9049. Mobile: 07831 802 598.

AUTHOR'S ACKNOWLEDGMENTS

Whatever understanding I have of the martial arts, I owe to my masters. They treated me like a member of the family, taught from their hearts, pushed me hard and never hid anything from me. It was Master Lai in Hong Kong who trained me for tournaments. When I was still a teenager Buddhist Master Lau Sau Hong broadened my horizons by introducing me to the arts of Zhan Zhuang, Feng Shui, Taoism and Buddhism. Professor Yu Yong Nian became like a father to me, allowing me to live and train with him in Beijing where he revealed the depths of Da Cheng Chuan. To Madame Wang Yuk Fong, and all the disciples of her father who shared their knowledge with me, I am deeply indebted.

Without the support, patience and trust of my wife, Lam Kai Sin, I could never have devoted myself so totally to this art. My three sons have followed in this tradition and have helped me experiment with new ideas as we train together. In particular, I would like to thank Tin Hun for his work on the inner architecture of the body and his research into bridge bearings.

Transmitting the essence of this art across the barriers of language and culture is not easy. My student, Richard Reoch, has devoted himself to this challenge, working with me so that this ancient tradition can play a healing role in modern society. Without our heart connection, none of this would have happened. I would also like to thank the many other students who have made this book possible, through their cooperation over the years in which I have studied, researched and taught in the West.

The designer, Bridget Morley, has really brought this book to life with her tireless work, the supervision of all photography, her illustrations and the great care she has taken to present the authentic spirit of Da Cheng Chuan. Joss Pearson, the Managing Director of Gaia Books, has continued to support me over the years so that we can bring the benefits of these arts to a wide international audience. Pip Morgan kindly edited the final text.

PHOTOGRAPHIC ACKNOWLEDGMENTS *Posture photographs of Master Lam by Paul Forrester. Photo montages 108, 112, 116, 120, 126 Michael Posen. Historical images supplied by Master Lam. SCIENCE PHOTO LIBRARY: 34 Dr. Morley Read; 76 David Nunuk; 82 Jimmy Fox; 118 Peter Menzel; 122 Bernhard Edmaier; 126 Ken M. Johns. 110 John Lund/GETTY IMAGES. 114 Graham Wren/OXFORD SCIENTIFIC FILMS. 152 Christian Herzenberger. 129 Ideel Reklame & Marketing. 2 Bridget Morley.*